Free To Move

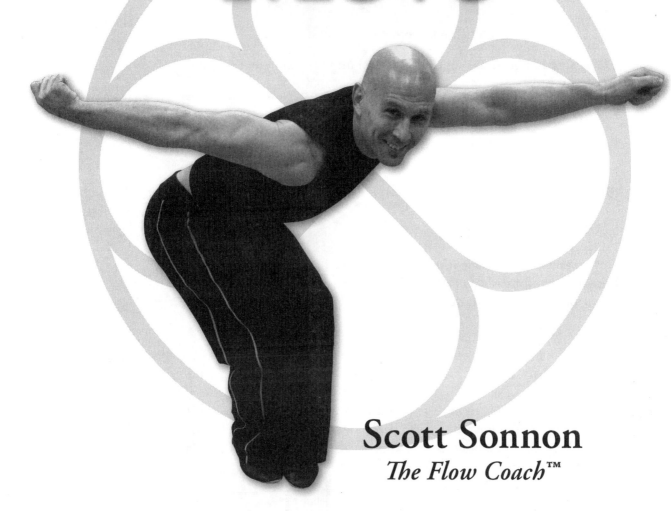

Scott Sonnon
The Flow Coach™

For information on Scott Sonnon and RMAX.tv Productions, please contact:
RMAX.tv Productions
P.O. Box 501388
Atlanta, GA 31150
Website: www.rmaxinternational.com

Comments and questions should be sent to: info@rmaxinternational.com

Intu-Flow® and Circular Strength Training® are registered trademarks of RMAX.tv Productions.

Printed and bound in the United States of America.

ISBN-13: 978-0-9794275-6-5
ISBN-10: 0-9794275-6-8

Credits
Editing: Amy Norcross
Design and Layout: Wade Munson • www.wadeincreativity.com
Photography: John Meloy • www.johnnydanger.net
Contributing Authors: Jarlo Ilano, L.P.T. and Kathryn Woodall, D.C.

Disclaimer
None of the information contained in this book is intended to be taken as medical advice. Should you have any condition that requires professional medical attention, please always consult a doctor before you begin any exercises presented in this book or any other source. Albeit the information and advice in this book are believed to be accurate, neither the publisher nor the author will be held liable for any injury, damages, losses, claims, actions, proceedings, expenses, or costs (including legal) that result from using instructions, advice, or exercises in this book.

Introduction. 1

    Ancient Discipline Turned Modern Science!. 3

    The Key to a Stress-Free, Blissful Life? 4

    The Secret Sequence: The Fountain of Youth 5

    Vibrance: The Return of Nutrition, Lubrication,
    and Shock Absorption to Your Joints 6

    The "Ultimate Challenge" 7

    You Don't Need to Be Athletic! 12

    The Only Impossibility with Intu-Flow Is Failure! You Only Win! 12

Spirit Matters. 15

Movement and Stillness. 19

Flow Beyond Thought 21

    The Early Years 23

    Ancient Discipline to Modern Science 24

    Soviet Peak Performance 26

The Perfect Fight: Zero Resistance. 29

Know F.L.O.W. 33

    Let Go. Let God.. 34

    Backing Up What I Believe In 34

    The Mantle of Emotion 35

    Healing Inside Out; Moving Outside In. 36

Grace and Disgrace 39

All Tonicity Is Conscious. 43

Higher Vibration Through Martial Art 47

Higher Vibration Through Athletics 49

    Linkage Versus Leakage. 51

Fear to Flow. 55

    Going Fetal 56

Fit to Flow 59

    Fitness as a Vehicle to Flow 61

    Moving with More Energy or Less 62

Complex Does Not Mean Complicated! 65

    Making the Mistakes of a Master 67

Degrees of Freedom 71

Finding Harmony 77

Mobility Expresses the Heart 81

Owning Your Movement 85

Loving Your Immobility 89

    Needing No Handout 92

The Problem with Stretching 95

    Debunking the Stretching Myth 96

    Does It Stretch Back!? 97

    Rubber Band Man 97

    The Stretch Reflex 98

    Flexibility Is Speed Specific 99

    Plastic Changes 100

    Health Risks of Static Stretching 101

    Short-Range Stiffness 101

    The Essence of Synergy: Range of Motion 101

    Mobility Practice 102

The Myofascial Matrix 105

    Snags in the Sweater 106

The Fascial Layers 107

Biotensegrity 109

The "Double Bag" 113

    Adaptation and Restriction 114

    Overcompensation 115

Crown Down and Heart Apart 119

"Wash the Inner Bag" 121

    The Progression of Physical Vibrance 122

Intuitive Training 125

Understanding Pain 127

Understanding Snap, Crackle, Pop! 139

Prehab, Rehab, Posthab 145

Aging: The Process of Losing Complexity 149
   The Nervous System Craves Complexity! 150
   Combined Movements: Lessons from Physiotherapy 151

Exercises 155

Jaw – Head – Face 157

Neck 173

Shoulders 195

Elbows 225

Wrists – Hands – Fingers 245

Mid Back 267

Lower Back 285

Pelvis – Hips 303

Hips 321

Knees – Legs 343

Ankles – Feet – Toes 367

Final Word 387
   What Is Your Primary Fitness Attribute? 387
   Mobility Is Your Very Existence 388

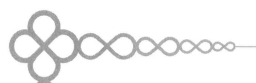

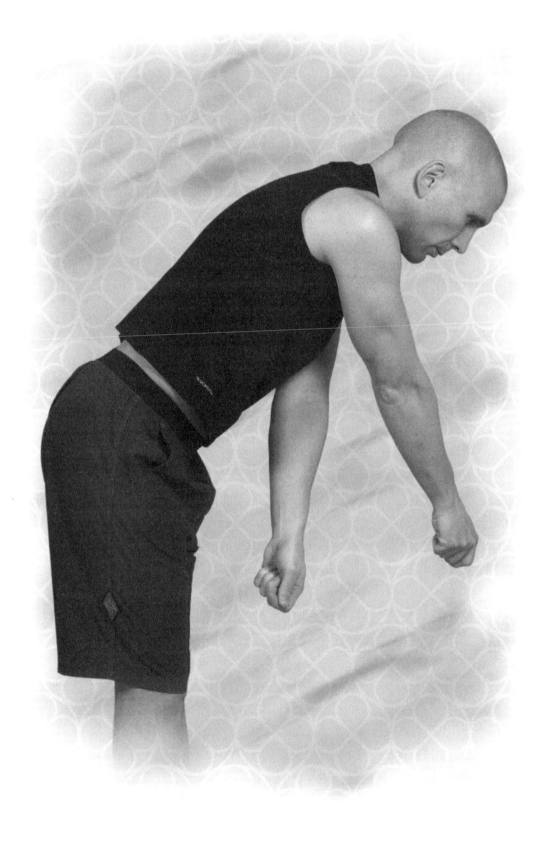

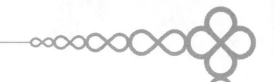

Introduction

*A*llow me to present the "Fountain of Youth": The Intu-Flow® Longevity System.

Are you Free to Move?!

End your concerns of poor health, illness, aging, and even death! Gratefully live a full century (or more!) of healthy, vibrant years through my Fountain of Youth — the Intu-Flow Longevity System — so simple to learn most everyone instantly feels the surge of potent vitality and crystal-clear awareness.

No matter how old you are, by moving each of your joints in a secret sequence for just eight minutes a day, you will be able to:

- Be pain-free without any strain
- "Turn back the clock" to reverse aging
- Gain graceful poise and effortless carriage
- Experience a perfect balance of mobility and stability
- Reclaim child-like vitality
- Bathe yourself in unlimited healing energy
- Enjoy true lifetime fitness without injuries
- Amplify your mental acuity and awareness
- Empower yourself rather than feel powerless
- Be your own gym without costly machines

Dear Student,

We're bombarded daily by one emotionally disemboweling message: As we age, we can expect nothing but disease and disrepair, incompetence, and invalidity. But you can be *free* from this self-fulfilling propaganda! How?

I shall reveal to you what I uncovered during my years studying an ancient health system literally turned space-age science. In the former Soviet Union's scientific think tank of Olympic coaches, special operation trainers, and medical scientists, I was honored as the first Westerner to "mind share" their technologies. These individuals had transformed millennia-old health traditions into cutting-edge longevity science for their space program to guarantee cosmonauts long, healthy lives, even when faced with the ravages of zero gravity (where all life rapidly accelerates the process of dying).

One of the men I studied with was a silver-haired monk nicknamed Porfiri. Though of an obviously seasoned age, he boasted of being 104 years old. Porfiri's seniority didn't prevent him from displaying extraordinary feats of strength, such as twirling a 140-pound tree around his torso!

Porfiri taught a Russian monastic practice very similar to the traditional yoga and Sufism I was taught — in its design to energetically align you with grace through specific postures, deliberate movement, and unique breathing exercises — referring to his ancient library called the *Philokalia,* meaning "to love beauty."

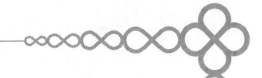

ANCIENT DISCIPLINE TURNED MODERN SCIENCE!

My Russian mentors delved into what has worked for thousands of years and distilled the universal principles. For weeks on end, I would be rigorously tested with exotic recording devices, which would bleep and blip as I performed the various movements I had mastered while training six hours per day. Soviet scientist and physician Alexander Bogomoletz said wisely, "You are as old as your connective tissue!"

In the United States I had improved the size and strength of my muscles, but in Russia I was taught the more subtle power of the tissue that surrounds the muscles, the joints, the bones, and even the organs. Though I was a world-class fighter when I arrived in Russia, I was regularly outperformed by individuals in their 60s and 70s — a reality hard-swallowed, but gratefully learned!

Numerous research protocols were still classified so I was not allowed to film many events, but one device recorded every one of the drills: my nervous system. I was forever changed by being required to master the exercises. And because of the learning disabilities and physical impairments I experienced as a child, I developed an acute sensitivity for movement, position, and force. If I did a movement once, I never forgot it. It was the blessing that resulted from enduring the "defects" that had dismayed teachers of my youth.

So, what were these exercises that guaranteed a long life of high-quality, pain-free movement? Whether you take my word or not, the basic movements were nothing more than learning how to move each joint individually!

My teacher, Russian general Alexander Ivanovich Retuinskih, sat me down on the very first day. Because of our language barrier, he sketched out how these movements were strung together in a sequence, and demonstrated each illustration. Through this game of charades, General Retuinskih explained that there are six patterns of movement that when done in proper sequence will spring your Fountain of Youth.

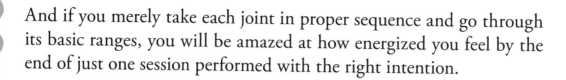

And if you merely take each joint in proper sequence and go through its basic ranges, you will be amazed at how energized you feel by the end of just one session performed with the right intention.

General Retuinskih would select a joint, press a particular point, and produce pain. He would then show me a movement and have me perform it. When he returned to the same pressure application as before, I would experience less discomfort. With each more advanced movement he taught me, the pain diminished until it was completely gone. And then something else happened.

When the "noise" of pain disappeared, a sudden whoosh of energy flooded into the local area; it then started to leech into the next adjacent joint and so on. By the end of this session, I felt like a superhero ready to take off!

Every one of those wintry, dark mornings, I climbed out of my rack in my skivvies to run outside and perform my breathing exercises, my postures, and my movements. And each morning more and more energy started to uncork, like a sluice gate was being opened higher and higher within me.

THE KEY TO A STRESS-FREE, BLISSFUL LIFE?

During deeper sessions with General Retuinskih, and my other Russian teachers, I came to understand the real key to this movement: Every joint carries a specific emotional component, so restoring the mobility in that area discharged the biochemical emotion-blocking energy. Each movement is accompanied by greater psychological clarity and stronger emotional power.

Movement is life. Without mobility, we are literally enslaved. So I moved the area of my back that had suffered a disc herniation. I moved it for several repetitions and then performed several squats to check my pain level and range of motion.

I stood dumbfounded. No pain. None. Full range of motion. Butt to floor.

Awesome. Completely awesome.

General Retuinskih smiled at the expression on my face. And then he rapped on his illustration to highlight that he had shown me only the basic movement at that point.

I laughed as he went on to share how the movements progress in a very specific sequence, which relates to the way we develop neurologically, to the way our spine and our brain evolve from infancy. Scientists call it the cephalocaudal-proximodistal trend. But the knowledge of how to take advantage of the energetic development of that secret sequence had remained buried in the indigenous Russian health discipline that I was given the privilege of studying from its masters.

THE SECRET SEQUENCE: THE FOUNTAIN OF YOUTH

The second secret to Intu-Flow involves a movement sophistication pattern unique to the Russian people. None of these exercises are performed on the ground; all are done while standing. And each movement unlocks a new valve of nutritive flow in your body.

Because Russia sits in the middle of the world, you will see movements that look like yoga, some like martial art, some like dance. However, it's the scientific, systematic recipe that sequences the opening of those energetic valves to restore nutritive flow to every cell in your body: head to toe, core to fingers, bones to skin.

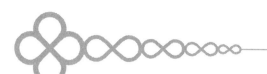

VIBRANCE: THE RETURN OF NUTRITION, LUBRICATION, AND SHOCK ABSORPTION TO YOUR JOINTS

The third secret to Intu-Flow involves the progression of the movement patterns from the simple to the complex, but in a way that you're never, ever confused as to the path to take. As you move a joint, you decompress the "stuck" areas, allowing the very fluid that provides lubrication and nutrition to reach these areas. You see, what the scientists showed me is that without movement, you are in a process of daily suicide. The only way a joint can get nutrition is through mobility, so if you don't move each joint through its entire range of motion, you are starving that tissue. No matter how good your diet is, the nutrients are not being shipped to the areas that need them ... without bathing the joint in healing movement.

> Literally, immobility is the aging process, which means that Intu-Flow is the Fountain of Youth!

You won't find one Intu-Flow exercise to be difficult or overcomplex. Within less than a minute you'll learn each movement, and when you perform it for five repetitions you will feel fantastic instantly. No, I'm not kidding. I've experienced this firsthand, and so have thousands of my students worldwide. The only people who don't benefit from Intu-Flow are the ones who have become so jaded by actual gimmicks that they walk on by the "real McCoy" and miss out on the instant, life-transforming results of this turn-back-the-clock energy-enhancement mobility system.

> No matter how tired you are when you wake up in the morning, these exercises will open your valves faster than anything you've ever experienced before.

Say goodbye to your espresso machine! Through my easy-to-learn movements you'll be more energized than if you had a triple shot, without crashing!

Due to the fact that these movements are so simple to do, they compose the ideal "sustainable exercise" routine for individuals who are part of the boomer and post-boomer generations (like me). My Intu-Flow Longevity System is really a "retirement plan" because you can start doing it now in just a few minutes a day, and the interest you gain pays huge dividends for your quality of life as you age — and continue to age without early interruption!

If you're an "extreme athlete" looking for a kick-ass workout, you probably won't be enamored with the sustainability of the movements. I hear you on needing trials by fire to increase your conditioning. But just like when I work with world-champion professional athletes such as Ultimate Fighting Championship fighters, your recuperative abilities are *more important* than your work because, without recovery, you're training is like a wound that can't heal. And the energy that you'll gain by performing the Intu-Flow program, even if only for 14 minutes per week, will give you the ability to train harder, longer, and more safely.

THE "ULTIMATE CHALLENGE"

Over the years, I accepted a few more high-profile private clients and designed and contributed my programs to professional fighters in mixed martial arts competition, including winners of the Ultimate Fighting Championship, such as Elvis Sinosic, Jorge Rivera, and Alberto Crane.

Teaching these extreme athletes is really the final word on practical effectiveness because they absolutely crave being tortured by near-sadistic levels of strength conditioning.

However, do you think that the best fighters on the planet would be interested in something that wasn't created to increase their muscle size? Well the response is a resounding and heartfelt, to put it in their actual words, "Hell yeah!"

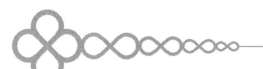

Read what the following health care professionals have had to say about my Intu-Flow Longevity System:

"The way that Scott Sonnon has interwoven and tied it all together is pure genius. As a chiropractor and medical doctor specializing in rehabilitation, it was very refreshing and inspiring to discover a system so firmly based upon good biomechanics and modern sports science. Seeing Scott move is pure magic, and his philosophy and approach to martial arts training are simply revolutionary. I have been practicing the Intu-Flow program daily for two months, and a problem I was having with chronic neck pain and daily tension headaches has all but resolved. I was somewhat surprised that as a physician specializing in such things I had underestimated the value of something as simple as working the basic ranges of motion on a consistent basis. The more I learn about Scott's approach, the more I am rethinking some of the things I have taken for granted in my career!"

– Keith P. Myers, M.D.
Texas, USA

"Intu-Flow has been a gift to my patients as a tool that is far superior, easily learned in small settings, and requires no tools. The type of neurological training that this system offers allows me as a physician to get positive results quickly, and even reluctant patients are won over by their own quick response to treatment. Intu-Flow explores your own mobility at the beginning of movement, your mind. The entire system of training is done in the spirit of healing. You do not work into pain as this initiates the panic/fight/flight reflex, dumping large amounts of hormones into the system. You are taken through your own body's movement patterns in a slow and safe manner, allowing you to pay attention to the small/medium/large problem areas. It is like going through the ABCs of your body. Once you master the simple basics you begin to add those ABCs together to form words, complicating your new movements incrementally, slowly speeding up, smoothing out the corners to mastery."

– Kevin Teagle, D.C.
Oregon, USA

"Intu-Flow has been a delight for me personally and professionally. I come almost purely from a health care point of view. Regardless of where someone is at with her health, Intu-Flow meets a person exactly where she needs to be and then lets her grow as far as she would like. It can be fun, done in as little as 30 minutes a day, performed in the privacy of your home or with a group, and allows people to progress so that enthusiasm stays up and they continue being active. The possible benefits to their neuromuscular system are vast, but the positive benefits of regular practice are certainly not limited to that aspect of the body. Intu-Flow empowers people to grow up and to grow old with grace and agility. Who wouldn't want that? Thanks for making such a great product available and affordable for most people."

Kathryn Woodall, D.C.
Kansas, USA

"I love this stuff! Scott's movement approach has brought excitement back into my workouts. I literally jump out of bed in the morning, ready to GO!"

Mitch Simon, D.C.
Missouri, USA
Cofounder-at-large, Resistance Training
Specialist Certification Program

"As a physician dealing with pain for the last 20 years, most of my practice failed to see the importance of proper sequential movement as a very important therapy for patients with pain until I came across Scott Sonnon. I have been wondering for years about the lacking ingredient that will make my patients pain-free for longer periods of time if not totally eliminate it. The breakthrough for me came from Intu-Flow!

By regularly incorporating Intu-Flow into my practice, even my personal knee pains and stiff back muscles got better. This gave me the confidence to incorporate selective movements for my patients in pain, which gave good results! Many more have benefited since then. The latest: a myotherapist in our clinic with a very bad back because of a long history of lifting weights; three months after Intu-Flow, he swore about the big difference in his flexibility and his pain had dissipated!

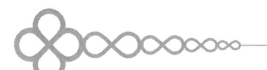

Now, all of my patients are given Intu-Flow before they leave the clinic, which will give them a better quality of life in the long run. Thank you, Scott and your Intu-Flow, for filling another piece of the puzzle for better and pain-free living."

Edwin Falconi, M.D.
Philippines

"I have been doing Intu-Flow for a few months now three times each week. I don't feel exhausted and beat up when I'm finished, and actually have more energy when I'm done! As a practicing chiropractor, adjusting patients all day can be a little hard on my body, so I frequently stop for a couple of minutes and perform some of Scott's movements, and it takes much of the stress off my joints. The movements are biomechanically sound, with nothing potentially harmful, and it's obvious to me that they were designed with that in mind.

Intu-Flow is the most rational and sensible approach to fitness and wellness that is currently available, because it restores joint ranges of motion first. By focusing on restoring and then maintaining normal joint ranges of motion and allowing your body to move more efficiently and gracefully, you'll be doing something that will very likely have the effect of healing many old, nagging injuries and preventing the onset of any new ones.

I look around at many elderly people who are hunched over, have a hard time walking, have joint pain, and have restricted mobility in their joints, and I feel determined to make sure that I never end up like that. Intu-Flow allows me to reach that goal, so I'll never stop using Scott's program."

Joe Myers, D.C.
Maryland, USA

"I am 63 years old, and have been working out since I was 15. Over the years I have managed to injure my back, neck, shoulders, knees, and various other assorted body parts as a result of bad technique, no technique, or what has been considered good technique by trainers, but isn't. I've trained

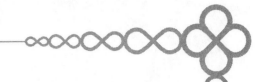

in martial arts since 1962, and have again dinged myself, many times, following the conventional training methods of the various arts that I've practiced.

I am a physician, practicing dermatology, but I have had fellowships in physical medicine, and follow the trends as they come and go. I was introduced to Intu-Flow a couple of years ago by a patient with rheumatoid arthritis. He was thrilled by the resulting decrease in pain, increased mobility, and dramatic reduction in the need for arthritis medication.

I purchased the DVD, and two weeks later my neck, which had hurt for seven years following a grappling injury, was pain-free.

I explored CST's many aspects, and concluded that I needed Scott Sonnon's teaching about 40 years ago. Well, better late than never. I am now a CST instructor, teaching a weekly class, plus a self-defense class using the techniques of Intu-Flow and other components of CST for attribute development.

I have seen in myself and my students, who range in age from 13 to the late 80s, dramatic improvement in mobility, balance, and grace in activities of daily living, as well as self-defense training.

With 48 years of training behind me, I find Intu-Flow the most rational, effective, and enjoyable form of training I've ever experienced, and I continue to explore the constantly evolving new programs available from Coach Sonnon.

Thank you to all the coaches I've worked with and plan to continue to work with, as long as I'm above ground."

James H. Auerbach, M.D.
New Mexico, USA

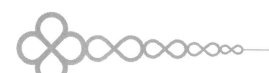

YOU DON'T NEED TO BE ATHLETIC!

What is the most surprising for a lot of people is that the Intu-Flow Longevity System doesn't require you to be athletic in order to perform the movements. Sure, with its help you can become supremely athletic. But unlike anything else I have ever experienced, you don't need anything to start. When you experience the incredible surge of energy from one of the exercises, you will discover this for yourself.

And of course, you have only one piece of equipment you have to carry with you: you! You are never "gymless" because wherever you are, whatever you're doing, even if you are bound to a wheel chair, you can start these movements. When I was speaking in Santa Fe, New Mexico, at an obesity recovery camp, nearly the entire audience broke out into tears because they just didn't realize that they *could* be Free to Move, if only they knew how!

THE ONLY IMPOSSIBILITY WITH INTU-FLOW IS FAILURE! YOU ONLY WIN!

And I have to admit that the most exciting feature of this system is that you cannot fail, you cannot do the movements "wrong," and you cannot hurt yourself if you follow the easy-to-understand instructions. Grace, poise, and the power that comes from them are *your* birthright, and these movements will help you reclaim them in most cases instantly, but in all cases you will be forever improving.

Even with just eight minutes of practice, you will feel like a human dynamo, pain-free, unfettered, tuned up, and revving like you're a six-year-old at the amusement park!

Despite feeling supercharged and pain-free, the biggest shock you'll experience with the Intu-Flow Longevity System is still coming. But of course, some people have no desire to "go for it" — we all have encountered those people who just feel complacent with low-quality living. It pains me to accept that some cannot risk losing their misery for the chance at this

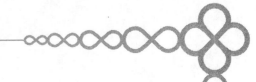

"bubbling bliss-itude." Regardless of whether this course may have given them a vibrant, long life, some just can't accept help.

It is likely that *you* aren't one of those people, so, mi amigo, I'm going to talk with you privately just a moment, since you've made it here and have had the intelligence to keep exploring your potential. Because you are reading this, I must assume that you're one of the progressive "longevity-preneurs" who wouldn't turn down a precious opportunity to gain exciting, life-altering results.

My 45-year-old Siberian shaman friend Vanya looks like he's 19 years *young!*

Watching my teachers in Russia move with the spry deftness of teenagers and yet knowing that they were 35 and 45 years older than me (and I'm 38) was overshadowed only by how youthful they looked — not just in their movement, but in their physical bodies! My Siberian shaman friend looked like he was still a teenager, so much so that when he took me on tours of the palaces to show me the rich history of his country, young girls would flirt with him. He would just wink at my dumbfounded expression.

That vitality directly relates to the regulation of stress chemicals through the breathing, postures, and motions in the Intu-Flow Longevity System.

Following my program will immediately start pulling back that old hand of time, and start infusing your every movement with wellness.

Join me in the dream of you living past your century mark in *optimal vitality!*

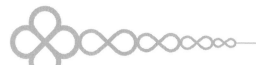

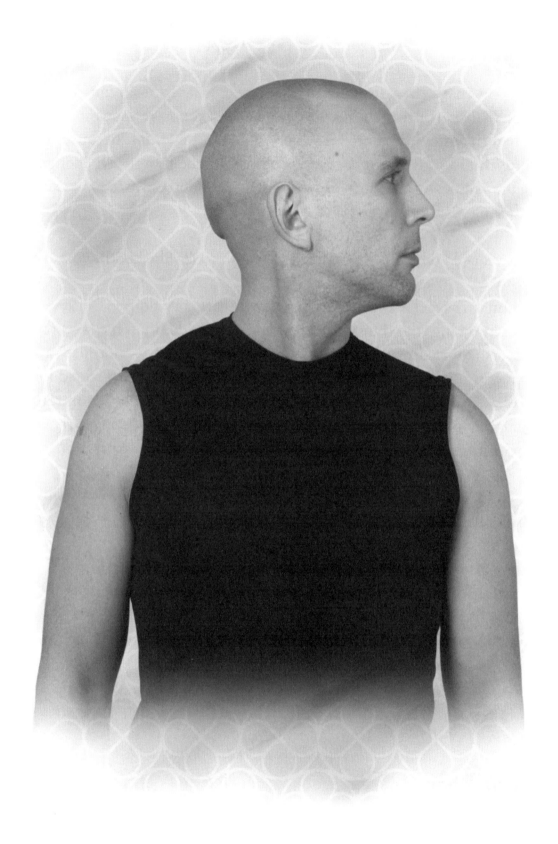

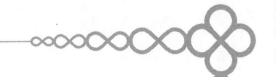

Spirit **I** *Matters*

**"Spirit without matter is expressionless;
matter without spirit is motionless."**
Dr. John Demartini

At a strategy meeting on our global initiatives, I was asked what was my ultimate mission, the underlying motivation for bringing my books and courses to more and more people. So I let loose …

We're at a war around the world and within ourselves between love and apathy. This One Energy, and the degree of its absence, has plagued the world with violence throughout history.

It is impossible to remain apathetic and increase one's flow; as our bodies become more immobilized, we devolve and become more apathetic. As we restore flow in each area, we release love back into our lives, and to those around us.

Physicists will explain that all things in the universe are composed of light, or energy. And all light is a frequency, a wave; each wave is a particular vibration. Everything in the universe is vibrating. Entities, including ourselves, are not solid, but consist of molecules vibrating at different frequencies, depending on the combinations of material from which they are formed. Vibrating molecules produce a frequency that can be measured or converted into cycles per second (CPS), or hertz (Hz). The human ear can hear between 20 and 22,000 CPS (Hz), so most of the frequencies of the objects in the world around us are either below (too dense) or above (too fine) our range of hearing. But this doesn't mean they can't be sensed. The very muscular tension in your body, each contraction, holds a frequency. Every movement sends a particular vibration out into the world and "sings" with it.

Different areas of the body all sing different notes, which, when blended together, produce a symphony as unique as a fingerprint. Idyllically, we would all be in harmony, but due to the constant bombardment of external and internal factors, we become fearful and brace and resist the natural flow. This immobile stagnation pulls us "out of tune" with our true song, fostering disease.

So, the goal of physical flow is to release our bound flow and restore ourselves to harmony by elevating our vibrance: The higher our vibratory aptitude, the greater our quality of movement, the greater the abundance of love in our lives.

You are not meant to toil the earth. You are not meant to trudge from one task to the next. You are not meant to be encased in pain. You are not meant to feel ugly. These are all examples of low vibrational experiences that muddy how we see the world.

Think of when you last had a migraine, or a head flu. Do you remember how it made everything seem lackluster and colorless, how you felt grumpy and snippy, if not irascible? The lack of higher-order movement, or absence of higher vibrational experiences, makes us feel that way to a much greater degree.

Now imagine when you were first in love, that first kiss on that first date, the first time you held hands in public, or even the first time your eyes met and you both acknowledged the harmony between the two of you. Remember how that made the world feel like a symphony and everything around you a gallery of beauty? The higher our quality of flow, the greater the vibrance with which we experience everything in our lives.

You are meant to move with regal grace. You are perfectly powerful always and already. You don't need to become beautiful. You must only share your beauty, share your vibration with the harmony of the world … through movement.

Flow is physical wealth. And you deserve to express your innate gifts of receiving and expressing your physical abundance, vibrance, and energy. When you allow flow in any one aspect of your life, it surges into all aspects. Open the sluice gates and flood the drought-ravaged fields.

There is a direct relationship between your physical vibrance and your ability to fulfill your dreams in the other areas of life — as I have described them in my DVD *Threshold Training* the triune of vocational, tribal, and physical, or as Dr. John Demartini expands as the vocational, financial, social, familial, spiritual, mental, and physical.

In this book, I will share with you exercises that restore mobility into your life. But these cannot be restricted to merely a "physical" experience, for truly there is no such thing as a distinction between the body and the mind and the spirit. These are all artificial conventions we use to discuss things that transcend language.

Flow is what we already and always are. When we are Free to Move, we gain the ability to step out of our own way, and allow flow to rush love unimpeded throughout our lives.

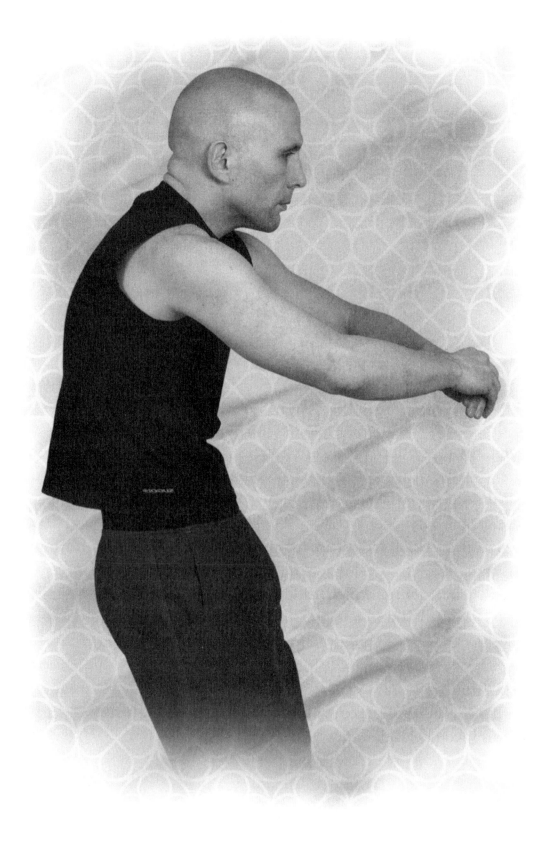

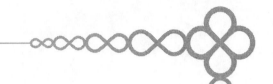

Movement and Stillness

II

> *"Music is the space between the notes."*
> **Claude Debussy**

All things in the universe move. Stillness is an illusion, a fabrication. Movement is progress, and resistance to movement is regress. Think of the "movers and shakers" of the world. Their motion shakes up, wakes up, the world.

Movement is life. The absence of movement is death. It's a law of the universe that aliveness is defined as movement, and death as stillness.

> From an emotional standpoint, and a physical reality, mobility equals freedom, and immobility equals slavery. What do we do to those convicted of crimes? We imprison them. We remove their freedom with bars, shackles, and straightjackets.

As I will discuss, we knowingly or unknowingly incarcerate ourselves with fatness. The tissue acts as emotional insulation thickening the walls of our prison. It requires enormous courage to begin the process of removing those bars. If it were not for the loving guidance of my teachers, I would never have become free of the walls of my childhood obesity.

> In this book, I will share with you the mental, emotional, and physical tools with which you can emancipate yourself from imprisonment you

feel, whether that be fat or pain or motor amnesia — even if you have forgotten how to move!

We will reclaim our liberty one degree at a time with a cumulative effect, which one of my teachers, Dr. Bernstein, named "freedom by degree." We will slowly thaw our graceful efficiency not by doing more, but by doing less. We can think of the opposite of stillness as noise, rather than flow. Removing erratic motion allows us to move with more fluidity.

Stillness exists, but we must reframe it. We must look at stillness as the absence of resistance rather than the absence of movement. Stillness is the goal, but stillness in motion. Through what my clients have called the "Sonnon Method," you can become like the eye of a storm: No matter how much things appear to be blowing down around you, you can keep your center, continue to move, and remain in flow.

Some have asked how I managed to develop this method and accomplish so much in my life in the face of such intense physical and mental disabilities and social and familial trauma. Reflecting upon the journey to the time of writing this book, I understand that it looks very logically sequential, but it certainly never felt that way. It only seemed like a pinhole of hope, an impossibly small escape hatch that was an incredibly long way from me. But really, what else can you do but climb? I tried giving up. You just sit there. Then what? Climb. Cry along the way, for sure, slip, fall, and start over. But really, there's only one option: Climb.

I feel blessed to have the opportunity to share this journey. The challenges I have faced are all compliments, because we're never thrown anything we can't catch. And all of those challenges were preparation; they gave me the chance to learn the lessons that others take for granted: how to see, how to move, how to think, how to feel, how to flow.

Mobility in its pure form is flow.

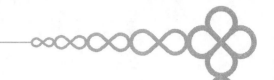

Flow Beyond Thought

III

"Exhalation is not the expulsion of air but the expulsion of ego in the form of air. In exhalation you become humble, whereas pride comes in inhalation. To learn this is to understand the movement from attachment to non-attachment."
B. K. S. Iyengar, The Tree of Yoga

In 200 BC, Patanjali compiled the Yoga Sutras, the "bible" that discusses Raja yoga, the discipline of harmonizing the body and mind often referred to as Ashtanga yoga. In the Sutras, Patanjali details the eighth limb of yoga, called Samadhi. Samadhi is the state of consciousness in which the subject (you) and the object (the world) become indistinguishable.

Samadhi is said to be the state of being aware of one's existence without thinking — a state of undifferentiated beingness. Patanjali names it the only stable unchanging reality; all else is ever changing and does not bring everlasting peace or happiness. In this flow-state, the mind has become quiet and given up its desires and attendant. Some teachers describe it as complete absorption into the object of one's pure, unmotivated love of God.

In his book *Autobiography of a Yogi*, Paramahansa Yogananda gives this stirring description of Samadhi: "An oceanic joy broke upon calm endless shores of my soul. A swelling glory within me began to envelop towns, continents, the earth, solar and stellar systems, tenuous nebulae, and floating universes. The entire cosmos, gently luminous, like a city seen afar at night, glimmered within the infinitude of my being. Irradiating splendor issued from my nucleus to every part of the universal structure. Blissful amrita, the nectar of immortality, pulsed through me with a quicksilverlike fluidity. The creative voice of God I heard resounding as Aum, the vibration of the Cosmic Motor."

When my students practice yoga, it is this state that we concentrate upon, the physical techniques of which I discuss in my book *Prasara Yoga*. *Prasara* is a Sanskrit term meaning "to flow without thought."

In traditional Japanese martial arts as I was taught, *mushin,* or, more properly, *mushin no shin,* translates to mean "mind of no mind." The expression draws from Zen Buddhism, referring to a mind not fixed or occupied by thought or emotion, and thus open to everything. Mushin happens when the martial artist feels no anger, no fear, no ego during combat. The distinct absence of discursive thought allows the martial artist to act totally free and without hesitation, relying upon not what s/he thinks should happen, but what s/he feels is happening.

Zen master Takuan Soho wrote, "The mind must always be in the state of flowing, for when it stops anywhere it means the flow is interrupted. It is this interruption which is injurious to the well-being of consciousness. In the case of the martial artist, it means death. When the swordsman stands against his opponent, he does not think of the opponent, nor of himself, nor of his enemy's blade. He just stands there with his sword, forgetful of all technique, ready to follow only the dictates of the flow. The martial artist effaces himself as the wielder. When he strikes, it is not the man, but the blade in the hands of flow, which strikes." (Soho, Takuan. *The Unfettered Mind.* Trans. William Scott Wilson. Tokyo: Kodansha International Ltd., 1986.)

THE EARLY YEARS

I spent my youth subjected to violence, perhaps due to my mental disabilities and childhood obesity. The physical abuse wasn't nearly as traumatic as the emotional terrorization. Long days and longer nights dreading the inevitable beating acquainted me all too well with fixation. My obsessive expectation of the next pernicious attack was far more injurious than even the worst multiple-assailant "boot party."

You learn fast that fighting back only gets you beaten harder. Running away only gets you chased down. And "taking it like a man" only causes the attackers to keep going until you are unconscious. Your only recourse is to "roll with the punches" — make it look like it hurts more while minimizing damage. Years of this "school of hard knocks" forged in me an internal change, most likely a coping skill to shut off the external violence in the same way that your nervous system shuts off pain to an area for an extended period of time.

When my concern for the violence turned off, the beatings became, for lack of a better term, less effortful. I won't say effortless. But they didn't seem as bad, and the emotional expectation evaporated. Less and less I catastrophized about what may come around the next corner. I don't know if I can qualify it as a flow experience, because I am reflecting upon it only decades later. I knew even in those darkest moments of my past, sobbing with bruises, throbbing with sorrow, that one day I would do great things. And it was that hope that pointed me in a direction leading to university.

There, I majored in philosophy with concentrations in Asian philosophy and German existentialism. This study happened at the same university where I earned a spot on my first martial arts team. The university team took me across the world, where I competed with great fighters. And it was the synergy between the object of my study and the subject of my experience fighting that allowed me to tap flow as a blissful event. Until that time, I had never truly experienced flow in fighting. But it set the stage for what I would later make the mission of my life.

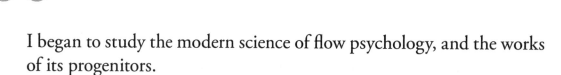

I began to study the modern science of flow psychology, and the works of its progenitors.

ANCIENT DISCIPLINE TO MODERN SCIENCE

In his book *Flow: The Psychology of Optimal Experience,* psychologist Mihály Csíkszentmihályi describes flow as the mental state of operation in which the person is fully immersed in what he or she is doing, characterized by a feeling of energized focus, full involvement, and success in the process of the activity. He identifies the following characteristics as accompanying an experience of flow:

- Clear goals (Expectations and rules are discernible and goals are attainable and align appropriately with one's skill set and abilities.)
- Concentrating and focusing, a high degree of concentration on a limited field of attention (A person engaged in the activity will have the opportunity to focus and to delve deeply into it.)
- A loss of the feeling of self-consciousness, the merging of action and awareness
- Distorted sense of time (One's subjective experience of time is altered.)
- Direct and immediate feedback (Successes and failures in the course of the activity are apparent, so behavior can be adjusted as needed.)
- Balance between ability level and challenge (The activity is neither too easy nor too difficult.)
- A sense of personal control over the situation or activity
- The activity is intrinsically rewarding, so there is an effortlessness of action.
- Action awareness merging (People become absorbed in their activity, and the focus of awareness is narrowed down to the activity itself.)

Csíkszentmihályi also notes that not all characteristics are needed for flow to be experienced. (Csíkszentmihályi, Mihály. *Flow: The Psychology of Optimal Experience.* New York: Harper and Row. 1990.)

The concept of "being in the zone" during an athletic endeavor is another example of the flow experience. Theories and applications of being in the zone and its relationship with athletic competitive advantage were the primary topics of my study in the former Soviet Union, when I had the honor of training with the nation's Olympic and national coaches in sport psychology. My Russian teacher, Alexander Ivanovich Retuinskih, suggested that "turning on the machine" improves coordination due to its efficient integration of the conscious and subconscious functions. Many athletes describe the effortless nature of their performance whilst achieving personal bests.

The legendary soccer player Pelé described his experience of being in the zone as follows: "I felt a strange calmness ... a kind of euphoria. I felt I could run all day without tiring, that I could dribble through any of their team or all of them, that I could almost pass through them physically."

Formula 1 driver Ayrton Senna, who during qualifying for the 1988 Monaco Grand Prix felt like driving the car beyond his limits, said this: "I was already on pole, and I just kept going. Suddenly I was nearly two seconds faster than anybody else, including my teammate with the same car. And suddenly I realised that I was no longer driving the car consciously. I was driving it by a kind of instinct, only I was in a different dimension. It was like I was in a tunnel. Not only the tunnel under the hotel but the whole circuit was a tunnel. I was just going and going, more and more and more and more. I was way over the limit but still able to find even more."

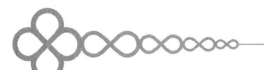

SOVIET PEAK PERFORMANCE

My study of peak-performance flow led me to Soviet Olympic coach Dr. Grigori Raiport and his out-of-print masterpiece *Red Gold: Peak Performance Techniques of the Russian and East German Olympic Victors.* Dr. Raiport, who earned his medical degree and Ph.D. in psychiatry from Rostov State Medical Institute, was associated with the prestigious National Research Institute of Physical Culture in Moscow. There he said, "We developed champions in every sport for world competitions and for future USSR Olympic teams; it was there that my mental training techniques of sports psychology were first used by Russian athletes." Suggesting that 80% of all athletic competition is mental and only 20% is physical, Dr. Raiport asserted that his techniques gave Russian athletes the competitive edge that earned them "a reputation of super achievers."

> When I stumbled into my university wrestling room to find the school's Sambo (the Russian national martial art and wrestling style) team training for the upcoming national championship, I realized that my path led behind the Iron Curtain. I threw myself headlong into the sport and devoured all materials I could, spending four hours a day practicing in addition to completing my university studies.

After winning several championships, I earned a spot on the U.S. National Team to compete at the Universiad (also known as World University Games, the Olympics for university students). As I traveled to international competitions such as the Universiad, I made more contacts, and began petitioning to be allowed as the first Westerner to train in the former Soviet Union.

> I refused to be discouraged by the impossibility of the Russians accepting a foreigner, and by the unlikelihood that they would accept someone of my genetic challenges. Thankfully, that tenacity led to my admission several years later with an email I will never forget.

In Russia, I fell into a massive think tank of research. Because sport was a political platform for the country, government funding created a flood of discoveries, tools, and techniques. The nation's special forces operators were its elite athletes and its national coaches. This fascinating collage of redundant talent brilliantly pooled the nation's empirical knowledge to validate and stimulate further research.

One particular KGB intelligence training director taught us the techniques for turning on the machine — a metaphor the Russians used for the emotionally detached, peak-performance attitude that brought them success on the fields of sport and combat. I quietly acknowledged the political programming that manipulates the sons and daughters of all nations to inhuman deeds, and by doing so allowed myself to study these techniques used to enter the "zone of optimal experience," which we better know as flow.

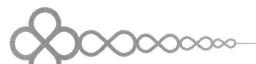

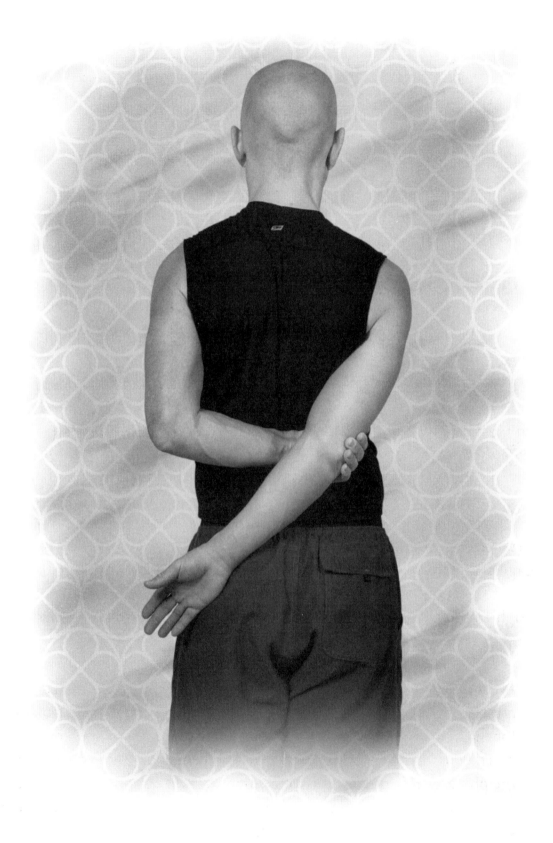

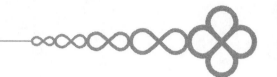

The Perfect Fight: Zero Resistance

IV

"Where there is love, there is no effort."
Amma

I've spent my life cultivating what I call the perfect fight. Imagine it much like the perfect wave for a surfer or the perfect climb for a mountain climber. The perfect fight is where the ego never pops up on the radar. No doubts, hesitations, fears, concerns; no attention paid to the lights, audience, or noise; no distractions; no superfluous tension; no inhibition. The ego is all of these things.

The perfect fight involves zero resistance. You exist inextricably intertwined with your opponent. The excellence that the two of you engage betters each other. You cannot improve without him, nor he without you, nor both of you without the event. Loving your opponent enough to give him no quarter and to give him 100% of yourself for your mutual development is the perfect fight.

I've touched it throughout my fighting career. Every martial artist does, but few realize it because they're on the receiving end of manipulation for the first 10 or 20 years. It seems so much like a physical event, when martial art is primarily an emotional and mental discipline by means of the physical. When you're "psyched out" by your opponent, he's created patterns of tension within you, dropping you out of perfection, bringing your ego — your fear, doubts, hesitations, insecurities — into you.

This may sound like a battle, and it is, but it's also a blessing. The best gift your opponent could give you is an opportunity to learn where your "hot buttons" are that can throw you out of your game. That's the benefit.

> You'd never know where these hot buttons were without him. You'd never even know the difference between you and your ego. Many people live their lives that way. They live their lives as passengers while their egos drive the bus. They react only with anger, frustration, rage, sorrow, et cetera. They don't have the opportunity to know that they are not those patterns.

Martial art is a seething cauldron, with a temperature not for everyone. Like my teacher Sri Mata Amritanandamayi Devi, or Amma, has taught me, not everyone has the same yoga. For me, though, it's fighting. The threat of physical harm demands that the ego be suspended. And once you develop the skills to protect yourself, you begin to learn how to step beyond self-defense. The fight is only the means to an end. The goal of martial art isn't the product (self-defensibility); it's the process: to suspend the ego.

> After you've developed your skills, you stop worrying about collecting techniques, and you start working on betterment. You start to get glimpses during your sparring. Your ego just suddenly evaporates in the most intense exchange. You respond only just enough to evade, not enough to fear — missed by an inch, missed by a mile, as the saying goes.

And those brilliantly quiescent seconds stretch out like years. They were among the most serene events of my life. Nothing wrong; everything perfect. It feels as if you stand snugly in the eye of a storm raging around you, though it kisses the surface of your body as it passes — intimately close, but impossibly harmless.

Those moments set the stage for the rest of my life. They were like a spiritual blink at the divine order: a micro of the macro. Those delicate moments of what sport psychologists describe as the "zone of optimal experience," and others still as "peak performance," launched my mission to bring that opportunity to others who were not "fighters" — to bring the process of martial art to everyone.

It required meeting an "earth worker" named Jo while presenting an Intu-Flow seminar in Australia for me to realize how widely accessible this state is. After having a late dinner together in Sydney discussing the "perfect fight," we saw each other the next day at my seminar. With twinkling eyes, Jo exclaimed how she had just had the perfect fight with her employer.

Her employer had been devaluing her contribution to the corporation because he didn't realize her efficiency level. To complete her tasks, Jo required a fraction of the time and energy that others did to complete the same tasks. Her employer had been fixated on the low number of her actual hours rather than the incredible efficiency with which she accomplished her objectives.

After our discussion of the perfect fight, Jo decided that she was going to go straight into the storm rather than skirt it and allow it to slowly erode her sense of fulfillment with her job. While Jo was in the midst of a meeting, her employer called her, demanding that she immediately conclude and report to his office. Jo could have easily allowed herself to be psyched out by this situation, but she realized that no matter what he threw at her, the best resolution would result. That's the thing about the perfect fight: No matter what happens, the conclusion will be the perfect solution.

Jo marched over to her employer's office and found him about to enter the building. Rather than waiting for him to settle into his comfort zone, she smiled and approached him, and they rode the lift together. When the two actually got to the boardroom, Jo opened her arms

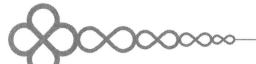

and asked the employer what he thought was the best solution to the issue.

He mustered his anger and threw an onslaught at her. But Jo remained emotionally detached. She maintained control of the situation in her posture, breathing, and movement in spatial relationship to him ... and resolved the situation to her satisfaction. Most important to her, Jo knows how she can reproduce the strategy by orienting on the perfect fight.

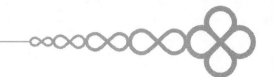

Know F.L.O.W.

*I describe flow as an acronym: **F**ollowing **L**ovingly **O**rdered **W**isdom. I have an unabashedly romantic relationship with the state, as I consider it the central focus of all physical disciplines. Flow doesn't distinguish between the head, the heart, and the hand. Neither should we. It is a unified experience in which our thoughts, feelings, and actions are one.*

When we "go with the flow," life becomes vibrant, effortless, and brilliant. When we allow flow to intuitively guide us, although we could never have extrapolated our trajectory by following the current, when we arrive at any one point, the divine order of things is obvious. Certainly it can feel eerie, but its wisdom remains undeniable. I use the term *lovingly* because we cannot force flow. We cannot even create it. We can only allow it to erupt from within us and surge through us.

> After not speaking to a former student of mine for six years, an athlete who had moved 3,000 miles away, I saw her walk by me during a Christmas Eve church service I had attended following an invitation from a friend's family. Compelled by some internal drive, I hurriedly excused myself and ran after her to speak with her. She was nowhere to be found. Three months later, I packed all of my belongings into my car and relocated the 3,000-mile distance to where she had moved. Four months after that, we moved in together. And a year and a half after that, we were married. If I had not followed lovingly the ordered wisdom of those crazy events, the woman of my dreams may have

slipped through my fingers, and I would not have become the man I am today because of her.

LET GO. LET GOD.

When you allow flow into your life, when you start to trust your intuition, magical events unfold. However, these moments of flow require faith, involve risk, and include discomfort. You may not know why you feel compelled to mention to the stranger standing next to you that you love her necklace, but when you surrender to the impulse, a wonderful conversation leading to a new job opportunity opens up. Perhaps you can't explain why you felt like breaking routine and running to the left path instead of the right only to discover on the news the following day that a mugger had struck again in the park through which you jog.

This same intuition lies within you. You may not be able to articulate why you feel like walking on the beach rather than going to the gym today, but submitting to the urge will result in greater energy. You may not understand why you prefer to perform twisting chair pose rather than triangle pose in your yoga, but listening to the little subliminal messages will always lead to increased health.

BACKING UP WHAT I BELIEVE IN

After a month of practicing martial arts with the Russian special operations military trainers, six hours of grueling conditioning and fighting per day, we were scheduled to put on a demonstration for the Russian government, in particular for the Russian Minister of Sport. To prepare, we rehearsed for many long hours after our mandatory training. While weight training one night late after practice, I felt something in my lower back pop. Nothing else happened, just that popping sound. No other incident occurred for the next three days before the presentation.

Our performance was met with roaring applause, and my teacher, Alexander Ivanovich Retuinskih, was awarded the country's highest sport distinction, Distinguished Coach of Russia, by the Minister of Sport himself. We returned to our rooms to bathe and dress for a formal dinner with the dignitaries and press for media appearances and interviews. A U.S. citizen training with their special forces was a major event, as I was the first Westerner given that honor.

I lay down for a nap and awoke in a corset of agony around my lower back. The slightest movement caused contortioned spasms throughout my body. Sasha, the Russian Olympic track and field physical therapist, rushed to my room to evaluate my condition, as did the federation's sports doctor, a Siberian shaman named Vanya. Sasha and Vanya put me through several highly unusual energy tests, and explained to me that either I could have surgery for the ruptured discs or I could address the emotional issues I was facing. *Either/or?* I thought. They said regardless, I wouldn't be able to walk for several weeks if not months. But my return flight was scheduled to depart in three days.

THE MANTLE OF EMOTION

I came to discover that facing the emotional issues was much more difficult than the surgery would have been, but thankfully I opted to brave the process. My insecurities had led to a structural and motoric instability in my lower back. Overtraining for eight intense hours per day led to the rupture in the weakest link.

I had been trying to prove to myself that I had the "backing" to withstand the toughest training on the planet. I wanted to show that I had the strong back needed to endure the long, difficult hours with the world's deadliest fighters. And I succeeded, at a dear price. The universe allowed me to complete the entire month-long event, but then required that I stop, lie down, and consider the long-term implications of my actions.

Thank God for the injury. It changed my life forever. The pain was the most excruciating I had ever experienced; and I knew pain rather well from my childhood. But lying there in that bed, I realized that I had to heal, not just physically, but mentally and emotionally. I had to allow myself to be fully mobile, and cease my desperate attempts to prove that I could handle any torture and not give up. In effect, I had institutionalized within myself the pattern of victim and victimizer, feeling that if I beat myself harder and still survived I was stronger because of it.

HEALING INSIDE OUT; MOVING OUTSIDE IN

I couldn't move my lower back locally at all. The slightest budge struck lightning into my nerves. But I had to move. Only movement can pick up the inflammation. But the inflammation was there to act as a splint to protect the herniated discs. And only movement could help the discs move back into place.

> So I began with my fingers. Slow circles … no pain. I moved my wrists … slight discomfort but nothing acute. I started to perform circles with my elbows, and the pain spiked. Back to the wrists with movement, circling until the discomfort vanished. Then returning to the elbows; the discomfort dropped under dangerous levels (about a 3 on a scale of 1–10; 10 being the worst). Following the same format with my toes, ankles, and knees, I would move closer to my lower back until the pain spiked about a 3 and then back away until it dropped under that threshold. Closer and closer to my lower back, to the neck and shoulders, to the hips, to the mid back, I stealthily crept in with mobility. Staying underneath the radar of the agony, the inflammation reabsorbed, I finally reached my lower back, naked of the splint it created to protect the vulnerable discs.

Chiropractors, physical therapists, bodyworkers, and energy workers all understand the emotional, if not spiritual, component of healing. Without any artificial distinctions between body, mind, and spirit, we must heal the entire being. Local issues in our body are metaphors. The lower back represented how I felt I needed to "back up" what I believed in, that I could "watch my own back" without anyone's help. The challenges I manifested in my childhood and the holograms I projected into my adulthood involved the very lesson I had not yet learned. I had not learned to love that greatness within me, and I overcompensated for my fears by "breaking my back" in the process. The injury was a blessing that allowed me to see the story that I had been writing all my life, and many lifetimes before it.

Moving my lower back, I began the process of restoring flow — physically, mentally, and emotionally — into the area. The Indians called this energetic area (the genital/sacral area) *Svadhisthana*, meaning "dwelling place of the self." The emotion associated with the second chakra is passion. If you grew up in an environment where emotions were repressed or denied, as I did, this chakra may be deficient. Signs of deficiency include fear of pleasure or self-worth, being out of touch with one's feelings, and resistance to change. Resolving second chakra issues lessens our "control issues," allows us to find a balance in our lives, and teaches us to recognize that acceptance and rejection are not the only options in our relationships. The process of making changes in our life stream through our personal choices is a product of second chakra energy.

As I will discuss later, physical injuries metaphorically call our attention to emotional constipation and mental stagnation. I had realized my lower back represented something far deeper than the stupidity of overtraining. And as I began the healing process of mobility, sending soothing lubrication and nutrition throughout the area with the movement techniques I had learned, I also meditated upon the miracle of my injury. That divine gift not only gave me the prospects to develop unique tools for healing and health, but it also allowed me to embrace my own strong back. I realized that I was not "spineless" and I had the courage to not "back up" when faced with challenges no matter how lethal or impossible. And because of that realization, I

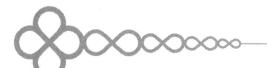

no longer needed to encounter that particular lesson again and again in my life, or across any future lives. It was done. I was healed. My stunned comrades watched me walk painlessly to my plane while my shaman and doctor smirked with knowing appreciation.

You cannot force flow, like I attempted to force courage by facing ridiculous risks. We must only acknowledge its presence, like the current tugging at our feet while we stand in the waves. Flow feels more like boat sailing than car driving. You can influence your course direction, but ultimately you travel where the winds blow you. The clearer that your intentions are and the more that you define your mission and passions, the more you will find that your sails are being filled strongly and sending you in the direction you need to go.

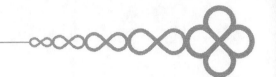

Grace and Disgrace VI

*"Thro' many dangers, toils and snares, I have already come;
'Tis grace has brought me safe thus far,
And grace will lead me home."*
John Newton, *Olney Hymns*
(London; W. Oliver, 1779)

I came to realize in my quest for the perfect fight that my moments of grace appeared when I felt the most Free to Move, light on my feet, like mercury across the mat. Equally, my moments of disgrace — when I fell from grace — happened when I felt backed into the corner, or up against the ropes.

Martial art for me was a way of reflecting this discovery from the controlled environment into the chaos of everyday life. It took many years of fighting to realize this. But our nervous system cannot differentiate between a true physical threat and an emotional, symbolic, or egoic one. We become aroused and defensive the same way as if we were in a real fight.

My best coaches, teachers, and mentors all explained one similar lesson: Perception is everything. One of my most brilliant teachers, Alexander Ivanovich Retuinskih, once took me for a walk along the rocky beaches of the Black Sea in southern Russia. As he pointed out the health benefits from reflexology that we gained by walking barefoot across the beach shoals, he asked me why I wanted to fight again. I

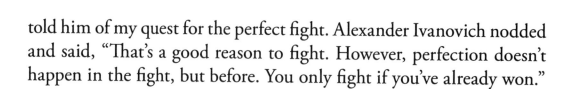

told him of my quest for the perfect fight. Alexander Ivanovich nodded and said, "That's a good reason to fight. However, perfection doesn't happen in the fight, but before. You only fight if you've already won."

Throughout the next month that I trained with Alexander Ivanovich and his fighters, he seemed to appear in and disappear from my attention. He would blip on my radar, smile, and say, "Graceful," and then disappear. Or he would appear over top of me, chuckling, and say, "You have again fallen from grace."

> *Flow isn't merely about physical vibrance but about awakening consciousness.*

The repetition of these attentional signposts allowed me to notice what I was experiencing internally whenever I was performing gracefully or disgracefully. When I performed gracefully, I was always exhaling or not yet inhaling (called the "controlled pause" in Prasara yoga). I was moving lightly, relaxed and fluidly, and I was having fun even if the intensity was extreme. When I performed disgracefully, I was inhaling or holding my breath. I was heavy-footed, tight, and jerky, and I was frustrated, angry, overwhelmed, or anxious. Alexander Ivanovich's coaching tool allowed me to see what I was experiencing internally and how that manifested externally.

> *Grace is a state of mind; ego is a physical event.*

As long as I held my focus on the perfect fight, I performed with surgical accuracy and beautiful efficiency. But as soon as my attention waned, and I began to catastrophize on how much better skilled my opponent was or how poorly I felt, my ego would enter my body and shanghai my performance. I'd tighten up, inhale, brace, and expect the worst.

Falling from grace is a very specific transition from loving to move, to wanting to move, to having to move, to believing you cannot. It becomes very easy to pervert our movement into something grotesque. We usher apathy into our lives through immobility by becoming disgraceful. When you don't feel like moving, consider the downward spiral of it. I know how hard it is, especially when you feel the physical pain of arthritis or the emotional pain of depression. But if we don't move, eventually we won't be able to. And if we do move, if we allow ourselves the opportunity to twirl in the exuberant dance of life, we release grace back into our lives, and into everyone around us.

Releasing grace into your life as a result requires a shift in consciousness. Since there is no distinction between your mind and body, you can do this through mentally reframing your perspective on a situation, or you can do this physically through mobility and breathing.

An exhale is an example of a shift in consciousness. As you exhale, you change to a more relaxed state; you slow your heart rate, lower your blood pressure, and release tension throughout your body. However, remembering to exhale and relax tension in the face of a crisis or emotionally arousing event requires daily practice of mobility. You can be as serene as you want in your morning meditation class, but spend the rest of the day with a couple of squabbling, crabby, sniffly, hungry, and tired two-year-old children, and remembering to exhale and not get emotionally aroused nears saintliness.

Reading this book is an exercise in shifting consciousness. After completing this book, and the exercises in it, you will have already implemented change in your life. It's like having a friend who is a chiropractor or yoga instructor walk into your room and start talking to you about posture, or a therapist talking about relaxing through breath control. Suddenly, you regain an antigravitational posture and begin exhaling again. Reading this book, however, gives you a much greater granularity of awareness, down to the minutest abiding place of tension, so that you can release the sluice gates on your grace long before they become dammed up.

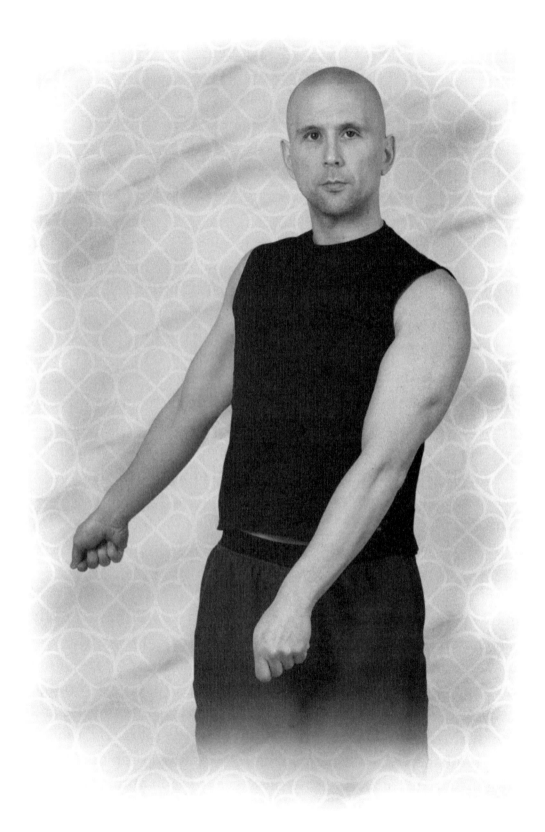

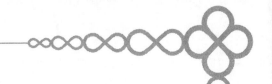

All Tonicity Is Conscious VII

"Your mind should be nowhere in particular."
Takuan Soho

*O*ne of the lessons I learned from a respected colleague of mine at RMAX International, Jarlo Ilano, one of the best physical therapists I have been treated by, is that all tonicity is conscious. If you are holding tension in your body somewhere, you are doing so deliberately, and you can release it consciously just as well.

All tension in your body is resistance: resistance to gravity, resistance to pressure, or resistance to force. If we didn't have tension, we would fall into a puddle of goo. My colleague, Dr. Stephen Levin, the father of biotensegrity, once described the human body as a "sea of continuous tension pulling inward fascially, with a scaffolding of bony compressive struts pushing outward." If we didn't have the animating force of tension, our very heart would fail to deliver our vital flow throughout our body.

But we can equally hold unnecessary tension. We can encase ourselves in a rusty suit of armor. And we do so consciously. We create it consciously, and we release it consciously. All tension is ego. We need ego to exist. And as one of my best friends Michael Gannon said to me once, "There was never a namby-pamby milquetoast guru; you need a hell of a strong ego to defeat the ego."

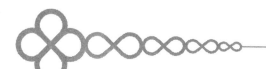

If you're holding tension, it's because your ego perceives a threat, real or imagined. If grace and disgrace are states of mind, and all tension is ego, then to have the perfect fight you must suspend the ego. You must release all unnecessary tension. You must flow.

I came to realize martial art is just a physical trick to convince the mind to adopt a higher vibratory frequency: to be more graceful, and less disgraceful. The immediate and traumatic feedback of being hit, thrown, or joint-locked tells you precisely where you're holding tension. It shows you where your ego abides within you, when your mind should have no abiding place. Wherever you stop mentally, you amplify emotionally, and brace physically.

Becoming mobile again, regaining flow throughout your movement, is only a choice when you remember how to move. Sometimes you need help to coach you through the movement, to teach you where and what to move. Thomas Hanna coined the term *sensory-motor amnesia* in his magnum opus *Somatics* to refer to the phenomenon that we can temporarily forget how to move a particular way because the cobwebs have become so overgrown from disuse — though as I will discuss, even athletes can cause this amnesia through overuse and misuse as well.

There are also more embedded issues. The longer you remain in a state of disgrace, the harder it becomes to move again. I spent most of my childhood disgraced. My physical and mental disabilities felt like an avalanche of incompetence. My posture slowly eroded as I hunched forward, my head dropping down, my shoulders rolling forward, my tail tucking between my knees. That, coupled with the physical and emotional abuse from those who didn't understand my conditions, caused my fall from grace at an early age. And I spent the better part of a decade clawing my way back up to release grace back into my life.

Along the way, I've had to develop very specific, highly remedial techniques for enabling flow in my life. My genetic hurdles, and the diseases I've faced, enabled me to create programs that allow others facing my degree of challenges to release grace back into their lives.

Martial art, yoga, and physical exercise are three prominent methods for consciously realizing patterns of tension throughout your body. By bringing these patterns to a conscious level, you gain the ability to release the blockages and restore flow back into your life.

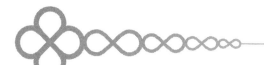

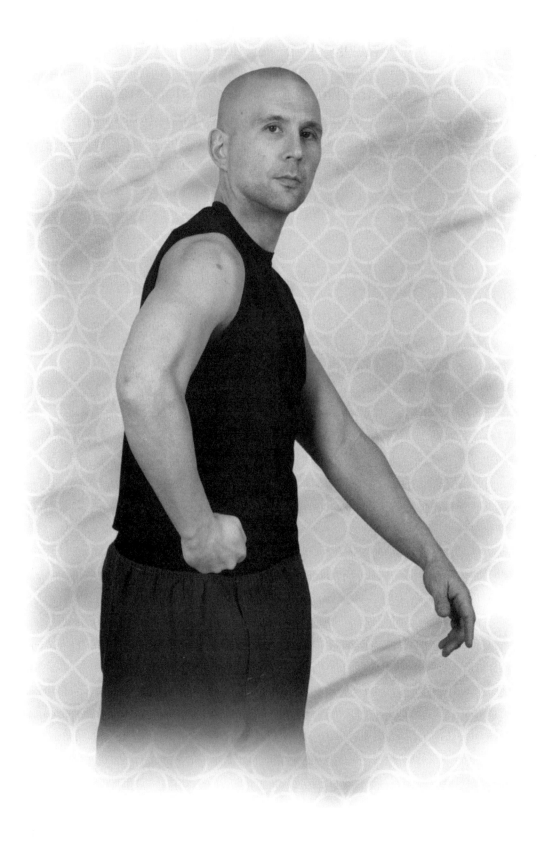

Higher Vibration Through Martial Art

In martial art, you learn techniques to defend yourself. But you always start with too much tension; you overreact and become emotionally attached to each attack. As you progress, you start to use less tension to accomplish the same goal, you begin to respond more proportionally to the force of the opponent, and you start to feel less emotional about being popped on the nose. Masters of martial art appear completely at ease, with the sangfroid demeanor of a monk despite the ubiquity of violent volleys flying around their head.

The internal event of martial art holds all of the secrets, while the external expression demonstrates the success of your development. The breathing techniques, the relaxation drills, and the movement sophistication teach you how to release ego when it abides somewhere in particular. When tension parks itself somewhere in your body, your teacher gives you tools to clear out the unwanted tenant, and light up the vacancy sign again.

> Wherever there is unnecessary tension, there is a fulcrum of resistance. Like a stiff neck will get you knocked out if you are hit on the chin, tension creates the opportunity for force to be transferred into your body. If tension exists only where it needs to be, to fold around force, and absorb and discharge it, then you remain virtually impervious to an opponent.

However, it never gets easier in martial art, despite how confident the masters may appear, because as you continue your path of

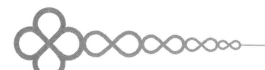

development, you face deeper and broader challenges. It's as simple as having higher-quality opponents. But more important than that, what happens in martial art is that to improve as a fighter, you must apply the lessons learned in it throughout your life. You can't be stressed out, unproductive, and undisciplined in your daily life and expect to become a great fighter. You can't compartmentalize efficiency. I have some of the world's best fighters on my team; all are extraordinary individuals in their personal lives who have used martial art as a vehicle for personal transformation.

Martial art tricks you into moving more efficiently and becoming more centered and composed, not just within the fight but throughout your entire life. You learn to move with grace in all things, not just in the little laboratory of fighting.

Mastering martial art comes in understanding it's just a path for that grace to erupt within you. It's not for all people. You can just as effectively use exercise or yoga.

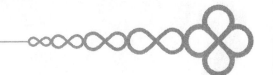

Higher Vibration Through Athletics

IX

*P*hysical conditioning — stamina, strength, endurance — like martial
art is another trick to convince the mind that it can manifest its dreams.
If you're unfit for a particular task, your body tries to tell your mind that it's
incapable. And as a result you feel incompetent, of less worth, and useless.
However, if you're fit for a task, then you feel competent, worthwhile, and
useful.

I conducted a private session for a world-champion professional athlete
named Alberto at a beautiful park in Los Angeles. Before we began
the conditioning, we discussed how tight and painful his neck and
shoulders felt. I asked him what was weighing him down. He replied
that preparing for his next competition was causing him significant
financial concerns because he had moved into a new home with his
wife and newborn child. His meal ticket was this fight. That caused
considerable tension, a reflexive burden carried on the shoulders
because he's sticking his neck out with the risk.

After coaching Alberto through the movements necessary to keep the
area mobile, flushed with lubrication and nutrition, and taking him
through the specific breathing exercises to recover from the effects of
when ego parks itself on his shoulders and neck, he remarked with fire
in his eyes, "I feel juiced up! Like ready to go right now!" I advised
him to use the techniques judiciously because they can just as easily
cause superfluous tension in a different direction. Grace is the goal, the
process, and the way. As long as Alberto felt Free to Move, the weight

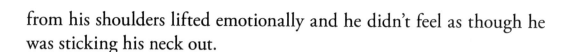

from his shoulders lifted emotionally and he didn't feel as though he was sticking his neck out.

I will discuss this idea in a much more in-depth way later in the book — how our emotions use metaphor to point out physical issues, and how to resolve those issues by listening and acting upon them. I use the example here to demonstrate that falling from grace is a conscious act. And just as consciously, you can choose to remain graceful. Like my friend Michael said, a strong ego (consciousness) is required to defeat the ego (tension.)

> *Power and the ability to express power*
> *distinguish themselves by quality of movement.*

Although weight lifting has been used as a form of developing power, the conventional methods use techniques from powerlifting (strength gain) and bodybuilding (size gain). Like a tiger felled by a swarm of fire ants, strength and size do not necessarily mean the ability to express power. Power, or vibratory level, is the higher-order movement that allows the small to overcome the large — like the sharp frequency that shatters the solidity of crystal.

> The expression of power initially attracted me to martial art because early on I had learned the ineffectiveness of the appearance of power, and the dangers it presented. Continually beset with violent attacks, I couldn't care less about looking as if I could defend myself. I didn't even find techniques useful unless they were effective and virtually invisible, since flashy, ostentatious techniques only increased how visible I was to those who meant me harm.

The moves that I found useful were the subtle ones: a small joint twist here, a slight positional adjustment there. Regardless of whether I trained with the Russian national boxing team or with Soviet champions in wrestling, Sambo, or Judo, the subtle techniques distinguished the good from the great.

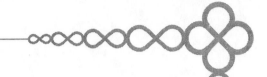

When I first studied with the world-record holder and champion kettlebell lifter Valery Fedorenko, I realized this was true of weight lifting as well. Valery coached me on very miniscule technical perfections — secret points of leverage rather than monstrous generation of effort.

The national wrestling team from Tajikistan demonstrated the same micromastery as they deftly tossed all competitors at world championships when we were in Kaunas, Lithuania.

Regardless of sport or discipline, what distinguished the masses from the masters was higher-order movement — greater vibratory aptitudes that we know as flow.

LINKAGE VERSUS LEAKAGE

In addition to the subtle micromovements, what allows flow to be expressed is the sequencing of movement. Many clients I train literally leak power because they have not linked each joint in proper sequence. A slight structural shift, through mobilizing an unlinked area, enables enormous energy reserves, much like plugging holes in a fire hose increases the stream power exploding from the nozzle.

When a joint lacks mobility, that area loses the ability to move. Basically, you lube it or you lose it. The lubrication squeezes out of the area and loses its shock absorption ability. Without that fluid, we lose our ability to sense (movement, position, and force). And worst of all, that fluid in the capsule between our joints, and under the (periosteum) cover over our bones, holds our nutrition. When you don't mobilize each joint daily, no matter how good your diet is, your connective tissue is literally starving because the nutrition you ingest is not being parsed out to the areas that desperately need it. You are in a process of daily suicide.

Each immobilized area leaks force because it cannot contribute to the summation of forces. Imagine a kink in a whip. The kink not only remains immobile, but it prevents the entire whip from generating any crack.

I once worked with a singer who felt her power was draining, as if she was losing the ability to "dig deep" into the octaves she needed for a new album she had been recording. She asked if I could help her, and indicated that she didn't know where to turn. Listening to her describe how much pressure she felt in making this comeback album, I noticed that she mentioned she felt like she had been "shouldering too much responsibility" for the recording, that she felt "weighed down" by how important this album was for her ability to bounce back with her career. I asked her a few questions about how she was rehearsing and recording, and discovered that for this current album and the prior album she had been sitting on a stool and somewhat leaning over to the microphone.

We went through some mobility exercises for her shoulders, and then to the adjacent areas where the immobility had been spreading: her neck and mid back. I also suggested that she ditch the stool, and make adjustments to have the microphone slightly above mouth level while she stood (to keep her slightly uplifted in her gaze and posture). A few weeks later I heard from her in an email thanking me for the Sonnon Method. She said that she had belted out the album with power she hadn't had in her voice since she was singing gospel in choir as a little girl.

Another client, an archer on the Olympic team, suddenly lost a significant degree of accuracy and came to me for help. As we went through the Sonnon Method together, she began to describe the new coach overseeing her performance. She described his style of coaching as tyrannical. I asked her how that made her feel. She responded that she felt like she was always forced to "bow down" to his demands, and that he wasn't happy unless the team was "groveling on their knees" for his approval.

We went through her technique, and looking at the position, I asked her if she had been having any problem with her rear knee. She said, "Not really other than feeling a little wobbly recently from sprints." She came to realize that the onset of her knee wobbliness matched the timing of the appearance of the new assistant coach. So we went through some mobility exercises for her hips and ankles, and reviewed her running gait so that it wouldn't deteriorate during conditioning. She called me from her dorm room a couple months later to say that not only had she reclaimed the surgical precision that had made her a champion, but she had approached the coach in private and explained how she had been feeling. The coach admitted that he felt intimidated being the rookie on staff and had been probably overcompensating by micromanaging the team's performance.

Although it may seem simple to see the issues objectively, some things can be entirely invisible without objective reflection: where you're leaking and where you're linking power. Because of my physical and mental disabilities, I had no choice but to meticulously dissect movement and reassemble it for optimal linkage. I didn't have the genetic gifts of most athletes, and my learning disabilities made mimicry nearly impossible. I had to consciously learn movement joint by joint. What I discovered through that process is that each joint holds a particular emotional and mental component. Only by religiously following my daily journal was I able to objectify my feelings and thoughts and see how the verbiage framed particular skill acquisition problems I had been experiencing. Three decades later, the Sonnon Method became very systematic. This book provides you with the tools to start experiencing it for yourself.

The next time you feel powerless, or not powerful, consider whether you are leaking or linking. How is your posture? Does it feel powerful? Do you feel rooted, uplifted, and ready to pounce? Consider each joint from your head to your toes, from your core to your fingers.

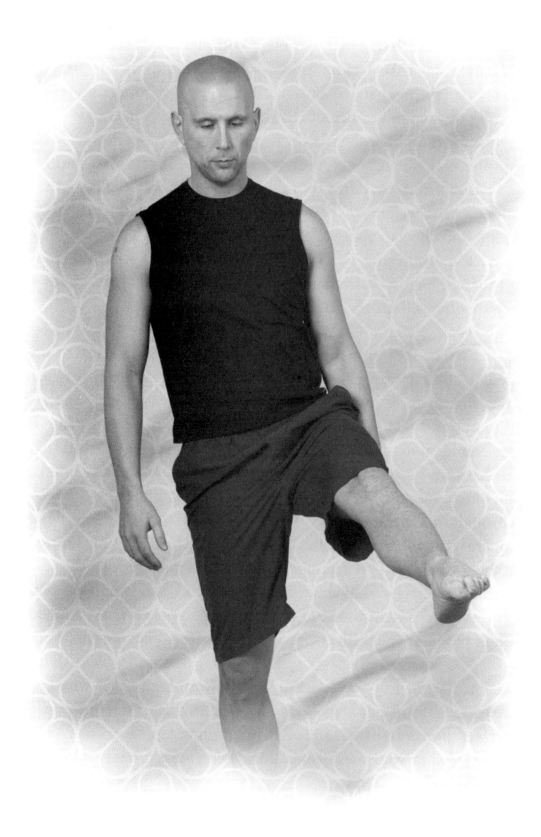

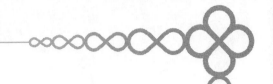

Fear to Flow

Many people hemorrhage power because of the tendency to overstabilize, which is a fear-based reflex. We inherit this biological gift to prevent us from additional injury when facing a crisis. However, this reflex assumes that we develop no survival skills.

Our nervous system cannot differentiate between a true physical threat and an emotional or symbolic one, so regardless of whether you're being chased down a dark alley by a would-be mugger or staring in the face of a belligerent employer who has obviously decided that his bad day is your problem, you become internally aroused for survival in the same way. Fear doesn't differentiate. It only knows on or off.

Something surprises you, some unexpected change in the plan, or you make some perceived mistake, and you feel the "whoosh" inside your gut. Your heart rate spikes, draining blood flow from your limbs and face and shipping it to your torso, core and legs ready to fight or flee. As a result, you may stumble, fumble, or otherwise lose fine motor control. Your pupils dilate to let in more light, which allows you to see much more, potentially dangerous, movement. Your breathing becomes shallow and rapid even if you conceal it well. This triggers your nervous system to tell certain chemicals to be released, which signals your endocrine system to dump jet fuel and pain killers into your bloodstream.

The hormones released into your system, although great if you had no survival skills to fight off or flee from an attacker, are a severe liability for operating in the modern world, for driving a car, for performing a sport, for negotiating a business deal, for public speaking, even for dating. From an athletic standpoint, you may have developed an amazing array of physical skills in your sport, but if you feel intimidated by your opponent, suddenly you shift from using your forebrain to using your hindbrain and stem. In an instant you lose all access to those higher-order movements as your central nervous system hijacks your performance and downshifts to reflexive movement.

GOING FETAL

Your shoulders elevate and your neck slides forward, your fists clench, and your knees shake; you may have to pee or vomit as your system tries to evacuate all nonessential baggage. You adopt the "primal forward flexion" as you hunch forward. This low-quality "gross" motor movement yanks down the vibratory level, and inhibits your access to refined skills. You just don't have access to them, unless you know how to flip the off switch on this survival reflex.

> This survival arousal syndrome (SAS), as it's known in psychophysiology, is a hardwired reflex. But it's specific to a particular degree of intensity of surprise or perceived danger. You set off this internal heightened-alarm system by being exposed to an unfamiliar threat level. So you can become desensitized to a coworker's bravado and practical jokes, but if your employer starts yelling to find out who's accountable for the latest foible, you feel fear. Fear is a difficult term for some to accept, but it comes in many forms: You may experience it as rage, frustration, contempt, sorrow, indignance, or any other variation. But your hormones have the same effect upon you: arousal.

SAS is distinguished from fear-reactivity, which is the myofascial (muscular and connective tissue) pattern of movement/tension that becomes conditioned through repeated bracing, flinching, clenching, and flailing. If you do become desensitized to a particular sound or motion, that doesn't mean it hasn't affected you. For example, one of the most common issues facing the many police officers I work with is neck immobility; the perpetually lifted shoulders overdevelop both the superficial and deep musculature attaching to the neck, limiting its ability to glide laterally and, in many cases, eventually causing it to lose the ability to twist and tilt.

The more that you allow specific patterns of fear-reactivity to be repeated, the stronger they become, the faster they are elicited, and the harder they are to recover from. Fear-reactivity also lingers after the danger/surprise passes. The more that you allow those patterns to be conditioned, the more permanent they become, encasing you in an armored echo of fear.

But as I discuss in my book *Prasara Yoga: Flow Beyond Thought,* this fear-reactivity causes more than mere physical binding of your flow. These hormones and chemicals create a pool of feelings. The mental thoughts that bubble to the surface from this emotional fermentation distort how we view ourselves and the world. Even though these thoughts and feelings are purely chemical, we identify with them and form our self-image based upon them. This insidious chemistry creates an identity crisis as we struggle with our own ancient biology to remain in flow.

As a child and young adult, I swam in a sea of chemical fear. I had no tools or teaching on how to differentiate myself from my basal protective reflexes. Like so many others suffering traumatic stress disorders, I felt smothered in the cloak of my anxieties. It took an enormity of love, compassion, and patience from my teachers, my wife, and my friends to help me peel back the onion layers of my fear and reveal my essential self. Now I realize what a blessing that time had been for me, as I can divide my life into two personalities: the illusionary chemical one of fear and the actual self, which lives in bliss. Having such a dual existence has permitted me to see the shell of fear in people, acknowledge it, and then speak to the essential self instead.

Clay, a drummer, was dealing with some obvious fear issues in his neck, having lost 70% of its mobility. That immobility slowly eroded one joint after another, from his neck to his shoulders to his elbows and, finally, to his wrists. The erosion now threatened to rob him of the primary joy in his life: drumming. Sometimes, we must work from the outside inward, and in Clay's case, we began with restoring flow to his wrists, hands, and fingers. With his passion restored to him at the site of his impediment, Clay felt he had the confidence to address the deeper issues, closer to the source. I would run into Clay every few weeks to see him smile, and he would tell me how wonderful he had been feeling in his drumming sessions. Each time he'd recount how he felt, he'd demonstrate how much more mobile he was. And each time he moved with greater mobility closer to that source: his neck.

Fear spreads, and like a blanket we sometimes must pull it away slowly and carefully, because going too fast, too close to the source issue is too difficult. But we can shave away at it, one layer at a time, and stay under the radar of that fear-reactivity until we have carved away all of the immobility.

Mobility, breath, and conscious recovery skills re-harmonize us at higher vibratory levels. We're able to thaw the frozen flow, like spring melting an ice-covered river; the current still runs strong. We must re-identify with that deep flow within us, and not be confused by the surface rigidity.

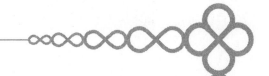

Fit to Flow
XI

"Only those who can see the invisible
can accomplish the impossible."
Patrick Snow

Many organizations and people have attempted to define fitness. However, there is a history to the evolution of the industry of physical culture — from old-time strongman stunts, to Olympic lifting, to powerlifting, to bodybuilding, to aerobics and endurance sports, to cross-training, to functional training. Each discipline's advocates have attempted to define fitness by their own discipline's goals:

- At the beginning of the 20th century, strongmen defined fitness as the ability to perform stunts.

- In the 1930s, Olympic lifters defined fitness as the ability to move greater weight explosively.

- In the 1950s, powerlifters defined fitness as the ability to move greater weight no matter how slowly.

- In the 1960 and 1970s, bodybuilders defined fitness as the size of the muscle's cross-section.

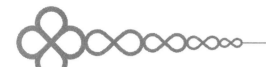
- In the 1980s, aerobics/endurance sport enthusiasts defined fitness as the ability to sustain a particular activity over distance or volume.

- In the 1990s, cross-trainers defined fitness as the ability to perform an array of exercises over time.

- At the beginning of the 21st century, functional trainers defined fitness as the ability to rapidly acquire and perform new skills well.

There is an obvious evolution of intention here, but in each instance, fitness is defined by its own techniques. Each definition has its own "benchmarks" (the term taken from the "bench press" exercise). These circular definitions have created what appears to the outside to be an industry. The definitions all still exist, but now they're either competing with one another or at least attempting to be housed under one roof.

I've been involved in fitness nearly my entire life. Initially, my physical and mental challenges dismissed me from conventional options. I just couldn't perform physical skills the same way as other children could. So I had to seek out alternative definitions, and as a result I often found myself investigating unorthodox approaches. Fitting in with mainstream definitions of fitness wasn't my goal. I was concerned only with what made me better, rather than with what made me more socially acceptable.

My journey took me across the planet. I studied with shamans and soldiers, the brain damaged and mentally ill, ancient yogis and new-age energy workers, elite athletes and underprivileged children, professional fighters and obese seniors. The cross-section of teachers I was given the privilege of learning from gave someone of even my genetic challenges the opportunity to progress and achieve what few athletes dare dream possible. But athletic achievement was never my goal; it was only the means to an end.

For me, there had to be some way to experience continuously that flow I touched in athletics. I sought how to use physical fitness as a way to allow flow into all aspects of my life, not just the physical but also the mental, spiritual, social, familial, vocational, and even financial — the seven areas of flow as described by Dr. John Demartini.

FITNESS AS A VEHICLE TO FLOW

To give flow entrance into all arenas of your life through the physical, you need to define fitness as a vehicle to flow. Some people must exercise to survive their situation, like the soldier preparing for battle. Being fit to work a job is a necessity, and many people make that the focus of their exercise. Some choose the lifestyle of recreation and leisure, such as the surfing culture, and any exercise they do is intended to extend the length of that lifestyle. And then there are the all-too-rare few who have courageously dedicated themselves to their cause, be it a discipline, a team, their community, or the world in general.

Much like Thomas Jefferson said, "We will be soldiers so that our children may be farmers, so that their children may be artists," the following list shows the progression of defining fitness with ever higher energy centers and intentions — from survival to work to play to flow:

- You can be fit to **survive** — to *endure, recreate:* The base level of fitness is much like the bottom of Maslow's pyramid of needs. Fitness is defined as the ability to continue living and reproducing. This type of fitness relates purely to your ability to survive a crisis and keep the species propagated. It's directly related to the first two chakras.

- You can be fit to **work** — to *perform, produce:* The next higher level of fitness is defined by its ability to function effectively and sufficiently. So you become fit for

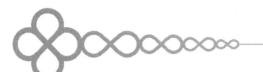

performing your job better, and as a result you become a more productive worker. Most people here concern themselves with the bare necessities and practicality of fitness. This level is related to the third and fourth chakras.

- You can be fit to **play** — to *express, enjoy:* Of the upper levels of fitness, we consider being fit in much more mature definitions, such as the ability to fully appreciate life and explore the world, as well as our ability to express our creativity through art such as dance and theater. Generally, people don't worry about their fitness here because they're too busy enjoying it. This level connects to the fifth and sixth chakras.

- You can be fit to **flow** — to *serve:* The highest level of fitness is that optimal human experience, its highest vibrational level. I say fit to serve because in flow the object and the subject disappear, like the Zen Buddhist monk who ordered his first hot dog, asking for "one with everything." To "serve" the experience, you cannot be in your own way, like the athlete must bracket her ego in order to interweave herself with the game's execution.

MOVING WITH MORE ENERGY OR LESS

I found that exercise programs didn't "fit" me because they didn't consider someone of my challenges. And even when I managed to fake my way through a program, I left feeling less energy rather than more.

I tried my best to walk among my fellow gym zombies, but because of my physical and mental disabilities, I was blessed with the inability to sustain those activities. Coming from poverty and from my mental, visual, and physical challenges, I felt that it was impossible to ever flow with the grace I saw in those inspirational figures I looked to for hope as a child. However, because that intention of flow is the most elegant goal of all human potential, I accidentally aimed directly toward it. I had no choice but to find alternatives that would generate energy, increase health, and lead to improved performance. I was forced to define fitness not by its basal levels of vibration but by its highest: that mercurial quality of poise that psychologists describe as the optimal human experience. I've written *Free to Move* because I felt a moral obligation to share what I've discovered.

So many clients approach me specifically because they feel absolutely withered after "working out." They devote all of their disposable energy to exercise, and some even dip into the energy needed for basic life support. The following example demonstrates a very typical sentiment I've found around the world.

An 81-year-young man named Paul and his beautiful wife, Patti, would always come over to visit me; and we would engage in some of the most wonderful conversations of my week. Paul and Patti had that sparkle in their eyes that only a full, blissful life can give. But they were physically damaged from years of overuse and misuse of their joints. Their doctor gave them the solution of becoming "more fit" and sent them to the gym. Paul and Patti were given the typical recommendations: cardio on the treadmill and incumbent bike, free weights, and machine cable resistance training. Paul would pull me aside with a smile and say, "Scott, let me tell you something. I spend about two or three hours every afternoon here talking to my friends." Paul disclosed to me that he really didn't like the exercises because they hurt him, and he often felt more tired all day long, rather than more energized.

The three of us worked together for an hour using the Sonnon Method to determine what was manifesting for them physically and how to reorient their "exercise" to empower the healing of those issues. Now, every time I see Paul, he grabs the nearest person within reach like only a gentleman of his seasoning can do and insists, "You need to

listen to this man! Before Scott, I wasn't able to do this." And he lifts his arm overhead, swinging it about like he's a lassoing cowboy. Then he points to Patti and says, "And Patti couldn't do this," as she wiggles her formerly frozen fingers with the cutest impish grin. Paul and Patti still spend two to three hours a day at their gym talking with their friends, but now they do it while performing their personalized movements. And every time they leave, they bound up the stairs with toothy grins, anxious for the rest of their day.

When you define your goal as a physical being to be in flow, you refuse to settle for anything less. The bland, tasteless fodder that you are served by conventional approaches no longer satisfies your ravenous hunger for flow. Fitness for flow demands that you accept no less than beautiful physical vivacity. By birthright, you deserve to have increased energy reserve through higher-order movement rather than depletion through lower-level vibratory activities.

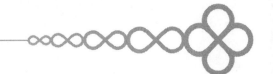

Complex Does Not Mean Complicated!

One of the most influential teachers in my study in the former Soviet Union was one of the fathers of modern biomechanics, Nicholai Alexandrovich **Bernstein**, *author of* Dexterity and Its Development. *Based on his early insights, a significantly unique outlook on the movement control "problem" emerged. In the past, research focused primarily on simple movements, believing that complex movements were inaccessible to most people. This is why we see the glut of ultrabasic "boot camp" calisthenics, isolating movements in weight lifting, and the pose-centric "yin" yoga in the West. Complex movements were thought to be too complicated for most people to learn.*

In my study, I discovered that complex movements are not complicated; only the method of teaching them can be complicated. The nervous system doesn't know the difference between simple and complex.

Dr. Bernstein created the primary goal of movement study in *context*. What's the goal you want to accomplish? Let's say that you want to hold a door closed. To "keep it simple, stupid" you would exercise with a basic movement such as a push-up. But the body as a whole, and the even the arm alone, doesn't merely extend and hold. It is spiral in its nature as a three-dimensional animate being. If you study human movement, like I've been required to due to my challenges, you see that the body is capable of so much more if you allow more complex patterns to develop. For instance, instead of just the push-up's elbow extension and flexion, add forearm rotation and you create the

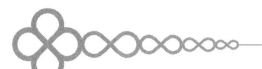

"screwing push-up," one of the signature techniques that have made my Method famous.

If we allow ourselves to "keep it simple, stupid," we'll soon find that we're stuck in simplistic stupidity. Either we move it or we lose it. And when we lose range of motion, we not only lose potential and options, we lose energy. If you get stuck in the belief that you're only capable of simple movements, you'll become right. If you enable the reality that you're capable of the most complex movements available to all human beings, you'll be right too.

What Dr. Bernstein proved in his research is that controlling multiple *degrees of freedom* (a term he created, which basically means "movement options") is no more difficult than controlling movements with only a few degrees of freedom. In other words, complex movement can be taught just as easily as can simple movement. Unfortunately, even simple movement can be made difficult and complicated due to poor coaching.

This is why I had to develop my Method. I found that most people learned in spite of the coaching, not because of it. Because most movement is taught to the 15% of people who could learn it in spite of the teacher, 85% must struggle to develop on their own accord.

When I was working with a neurobehavioral clinic teaching movement to brain-damaged and mentally ill children, I had the privilege of working with one particular boy named David, who suffered from Asperger's Disorder, which is a variant of autism. David's only connection to reality was through long-standing relationships, such as with his mother, and through "entertainment wrestling." He watched "pro wrestling" throughout the day on video, knew every wrestler's name, and could recount every move and match.

Due to David's large size, no one ever bothered to move with him; they considered his lack of motor control to be a hazard. The psychologist with whom I collaborated theorized that increasing his motor control rather than immobilizing it through avoidance would be much healthier and beneficial to David. So we decided that David and I would act out matches he'd watched after he learned basic techniques, including and primarily how to fall and how to pretend to throw. David understood that it was entertainment and not actual wrestling.

In the first session, I was impressed by David's enthusiasm because he was mostly disconnected socially. I worked with him on how to exhale when he fell. I taught him how to move his body so that I could fall over him and we could make it look to the "audience" like he threw me very high into the air. His movements were very jerky when we began, but over several months they became very fluid. David was frustrated at times, and there were moments when he used too much force, but my background allowed me to help him become calm and learn how to use "just enough" force for the task.

If you're familiar with autism, you'll know how monumental David's development was. When we began, David extended his hand upon his mother's request, and I shook his disengaged grip while he looked up and away. After several months of moving together, when we said goodbye for the final time, David looked me in the eyes, smiled, and squeezed my hand when he shook it. If you understand the disorder, this story will bring tears to your eyes as it did me and the doctor.

MAKING THE MISTAKES OF A MASTER

Dr. **Bernstein** explained that when we encounter an unfamiliar task we "freeze" the amount of movement required to accomplish the goal. In other words, our nervous system removes potential (degrees of) freedom so that there are fewer options to err. You can think of this like a hotel freezing a certain amount on your credit card when you reserve a room. It's still your money, but you can't use it right away.

Your nervous system looks at a complex skill and removes the unnecessary movement that could cause you to fail to perform the skill; your nervous system makes the complex skill into a simple one. After repetition though, you "thaw" that frozen movement potential and regain all of those potential degrees of freedom because you're in less danger of movement error. With practice, your nervous system doesn't worry about greater potential for error because the skill is very familiar to you.

Remember when you first learned a new skill and you were all fumbly and jumbly? Like when you first learned to ride a bike, you used way to much muscle, grew way too tired, and felt like a bull in a china shop crashing into everything within reach. But once you mastered riding a bike, you took your hands off the handlebars and steered with your knees, and even with just your hips. You could whistle a tune and even hold a bag of groceries while riding.

Imagine a young child watching us riding a bike like this. She looks at you and thinks, *Wow! I want to be able to do all of those tricks!* But she jumps on the bike and crashes right over the other side when she tries to lift one hand off the handlebar. There's nothing wrong with her mistakes. We all make those beginner mistakes. Failure is 99% of success. Unfortunately, in a society where everyone must be a winner, there is no room for failures. As a result, kids and adults are terrified to make mistakes, and thus there is a very slow process, if not a dead halt, imposed on learning new skills or even refining current ones.

> *The problem that the little girl had wasn't that she made the mistakes of a beginner, but rather that she tried to make the mistakes of a master.*

It would be impossible for you to carry a bag of groceries in one hand, peddle a bicycle, and wave to your neighbor with your other hand when you first learned to ride. All of that extraneous movement had been frozen so that the actual skill was simple for the nervous system to learn. That's why you feel so rigid and gross when learning a new skill: Your nervous system has removed all of the superfluous movement so that you can concentrate on what matters. You become fumbly and jumbly because it helps you make fewer unnecessary errors so you can focus on the beneficial, mandatory mistakes — those of the beginner.

However, once you mastered the skill of riding a bike, all of that extra movement "thawed" and you were able to hold the bag, wave to your friend, and pay little attention to riding the bike. The beginner can't make the mistakes of a master because the movement isn't available; the account is still frozen.

Practice thaws frozen freedom. And perfect practice melts it much more rapidly. Repetition of new skills makes you feel like you're gaining more movement, because you are.

I once had the opportunity to perform at the Bolshoy Theater under the tutelage of the famous Cossack dancer and coach Alexander Medved. "Sasha" moved like an acrobatic gazelle, effortlessly and powerfully. For weeks he tried to teach me a particular basic hand-balancing stunt. And every session, all I could think about was the advanced version he performed, which looked like a one-handed lateral planche — and appeared to defy all the laws of physics. Whenever we'd practice, I'd work on the advanced version with abysmal results.

Sasha finally spied my lack of attention to the basic technique and came over, chuckling. He asked me what I was hoping to accomplish. Sheepishly, I admitted that I wanted to learn the advanced variation rather than the basic stunt. Ever ready with a poignant retort, Sasha responded that "the advanced is within the basic — a deeper understanding of it, not a different technique at all."

Years and years of practicing the basics gave him the timing and rhythm to pull off the advanced variation. The extensive practice thawed the

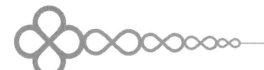

degrees of freedom so that he could make the mistakes of a master, which in martial art is known as "transcending the basics."

Sasha then spelled this out for me in movement by demonstrating the motor progression of the basic to the advanced.

Like a glacier, my flow had remained encased in rigidity because I did not thaw the ice through practicing the basics.

Months later, after our performance at the Bolshoy Theater, Sasha gave me what was considered high praise: He invited me to banya with him and the other coaches. There, he joked with me about how I needed to practice the basics of vodka drinking since it was such a staple of their health and dance.

The illusion of shortcuts comes from having new movement thaw after extensive practice and the mandatory failures. Once you acquire the new skill, all of that new movement allows you to increase your reaction speed and decrease your movement time. But no one ever learned a skill masterfully from the get-go. The mistakes of a master happen only through daily practice. Over time, with practice, patience, and determination, you will thaw your movement, and restore flow to the formerly frozen river.

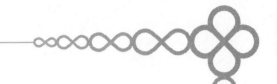

Degrees of Freedom

"Problems are messages"
Shakti Gawain

*D*r. Bernstein's notion of degrees of freedom left an indelible mark upon me. Because of my dyslexia, comprehending movement in the planes was difficult. It was cognitive based; you had to think of which plane you traveled through. With Dr. Bernstein's model, you needed to know only your movement. This kinesthetic basis for movement allowed me to excel and overcome the mental disabilities I had been formally assigned.

It allowed me to surpass even genetically "fully able" athletes because my mental wiring wasn't restricted in the conventional directional sense of right/left, front/back, top/bottom. But only when I started speaking internationally did I feel its full impact.

Years ago in Gothenburg, I presented a workshop to a group of Norwegians, Danes, Finns, and Swedes on my Method. They all spoke English, so we didn't have a language barrier. However, 80% of all communication is nonverbal, and the apparent silence of their body language screamed volumes.

Each culture expresses itself with particular patterns of movement. For example, males in the United States have little to no hip mobility, as represented in some of the endemic dances: line and square dancing.

Compare this with the fluid hip mobility of males in Latin America, where salsa and mamba dominate the indigenous movement. However, these men have limited shoulder mobility due to the dances' required firmness. Every country/region I presented in had its own uniqueness, and Northern Europe was no exception.

As the participants practiced the exercises, the language of movement began to weave its tale. Human movement potential, flow, is universal. The desperation lifted from the eyes of the military operators in between missions, and they began to work through the movements with greater ease. The seriousness faded from those whose livelihood depended upon increased job performance, and they started to have fun with the drills. And then there were some for whom even the enjoyment melted into a pure state of flow, where object and subject became indecipherable.

After several years of working with Scandinavian clients, I understand better the subtleties of their body language, as contrasted with the much louder gesticulations of people in the United States. But that week I learned the direct relationship between improved quality of movement and the elevation of vibrational level — from survival to work to play to flow.

Thawing degrees of freedom releases your energetic currency. With greater movement potential, you have more energy not only physiologically but emotionally and mentally as well. Think of the last time you experienced intense pain, fear, or anxiety — how it drained you of your emotional reserves and mental stamina. Now, remember what you felt like when that pain, fear, or anxiety lifted. You felt more than physical reprieve. You felt elation; you felt as if you had been lifted up. You felt "good vibrations."

This is one of the primary problems with conventional exercise approaches. If you allow yourself to move at lower levels of vibration, you reinforce and/or condition yourself to remain at those lower

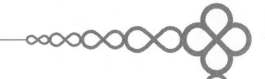

vibratory levels. This is why a good yoga, tai chi, Alexander, Qigong, or Feldenkrais session can make you feel more energy than when you started, even though you exerted yourself quite thoroughly. It's also why a bodybuilding, powerlifting, or aerobics class often makes you feel drained, listless, and even angry; it robs you of energy.

From a scientific standpoint, conventional fitness approaches wrench out the precious life fluid from between your joints and around your bones and muscles. Without the nutrition and lubrication within your joints and around your bones, each step, each movement, lacks the ability to absorb shock. And as a result it transfers cumulative microtrauma to your body. The compression causes your vertebral discs to eventually become dry and brittle, and causes your joints to eventually become wracked with arthritic pain. The postural distortions lead to impingement of nerve clusters and crush the organs when they should be floating in an effortless nest of connective tissue.

These are only the negatives, however. It is not the absence of their pathologies that creates flow. These examples represent only the low-quality life of pain, injury, and disease that results from immobility.

Mobility involves so much more than the absence of pathology. It enables the high-energy exuberance that you see in all too few people who just radiate with effervescence. When you remove obstructions, the restored flow channels a sum total energy reserve enormously greater than that obtained from merely the removal of pain or the healing of injuries and disease.

You become a human dynamo, spinning faster and faster with higher and higher frequencies and throwing wave after wave of energy upon everyone in your wake. A great Sufi master named Mushtaq once taught me the hidden meanings behind the "Five Tibetans," an ancient rejuvenation technique that has long been credited with giving individuals the ability to maintain youthfulness and vitality and to reverse the aging process. Its five movements correspond to each of

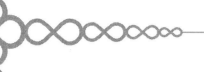

the five chakras in Tibetan philosophy, and stimulate the energy flow within and throughout each. But Mushtaq pointed out that it wasn't the movements but the conscious intent of increasing mobility in stagnated areas that held unlimited energetic potential.

At a workshop I conducted in San Francisco, Mushtaq advised me by observing my presentation. During exercises, he encouraged me to look at the movements I was teaching from an energetic standpoint rather than merely a motoric one, much like the Siberian shaman Vanya taught me in Saint Petersburg, Russia, years prior. And in looking at the patterns of immobility, I saw patterns of energy vortices appear.

Throughout my childhood I had intuited viscous points of sluggishness in my movement, which limited my ability to acquire a new skill. Unknowingly, my exploration into "vibration technology" in the former Soviet Union, and "vibration exercise" in disciplines such as Zdorovye (the indigenous Slavic health discipline), Indian Hatha yoga, and the Five Tibetans, helped me decongest those areas of immobility within myself.

Whenever I helped clients, I just "knew" their areas of immobility by listening to them speak, watching them gesticulate, and feeling them move. The genetic challenges I faced forced me to develop my intuition because I couldn't learn skills in the same way that normal people take for granted. The disciplines I learned gave me a movement palette with which to unlock a particular stagnation point. All of that background congealed for me, like a crystallization point, when I studied Dr. Bernstein's notion of degrees of freedom. This direct emotional and mental energy relationship with increased physical mobility formed the basis of the Sonnon Method.

David is a world-famous fiddler, a national-champion martial artist, and a law student in Scotland. After a workshop I taught in Glasgow, David asked me what I thought he should be concentrating his Circular Strength Training (CST) practice on. We discussed his background and current situation. He had been feeling incredible pressure from one of his teachers, an unethical individual who surrounded David in a web of guilt and deceit. David felt isolated, stifled, and depressed.

This emotional turmoil manifested in him as a mid-back, shoulder, and neck fixation. Using my Method, David worked on several movements to "release his heart and open his throat." I received an email from David two months later that updated me on his progress. During a meeting with his teacher, David told him that he was moving on because he felt limited. Despite threats, David remained centered and was able to express his joyful solidarity and leave. Even across an email message, I could feel the incredibly generative release, the empowered confidence that he experienced by reclaiming his independent soulfulness. David's mobility enabled his courage, which affirmed a higher vibratory state, and he became invisible to the aggressions of his former teacher.

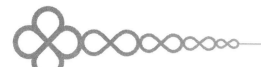

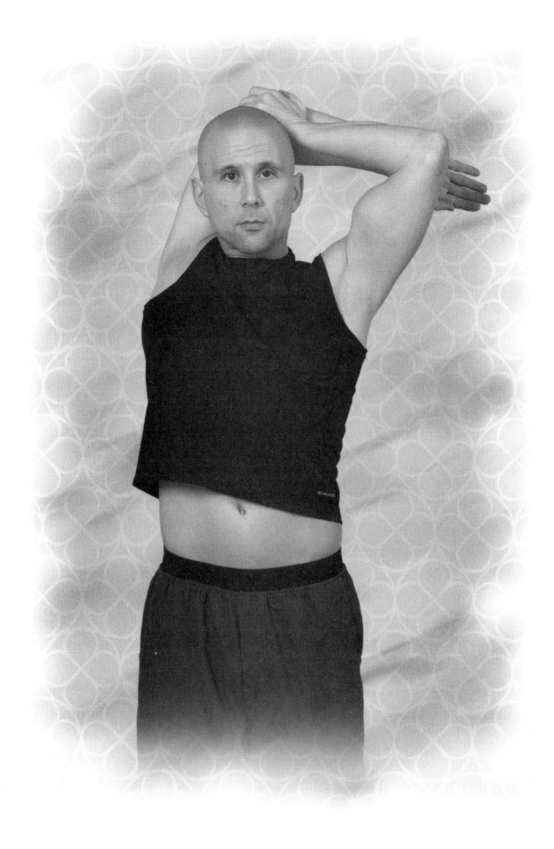

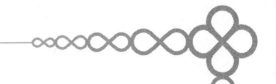

Finding Harmony

"As I have said, the first thing is to be honest with yourself. You can never have an impact on society if you have not changed yourself ... Great peacemakers are all people of integrity, of honesty, but humility. If you want to make peace with your enemy, you have to work with your enemy. Then he becomes your partner."

Nelson Mandela

Many cultures, such as Indian and Tibetan, believe that certain sounds, such as the cosmic Aum, retune the mind, body, and spirit. Sounds, or chants, are used to correct imbalances on all levels of being using a method known as "sympathetic resonance and entrainment." For example, if you took two tuning forks of the same note, held them close to each other, and struck one of them, the other would begin to ring! The sound waves from the struck tuning fork travel through the air and activate the other tuning fork, resulting in a sympathetic resonance.

Movement is no different, though its frequency is one most people cannot hear with their ears. As a result of being legally blind and suffering Thygeson's disease, I have been forced to listen rather than look. What a blessing it has been because those challenges allowed me to listen to the chorus of movement around me. It allowed me to hear the discord in my opponent's motion, and instead of fighting it with greater "noise" I blended with it, creating harmony out of what would have been combat.

When you're immobile, understanding the symphony of movement is as difficult as comprehending how tastes "can look like a painting masterpiece; certain strokes with certain colors just pop," as one award-winning chef in Portland named Sara described them to me. But you can feel this immediately, when you inadvertently perform the right movement. You don't even need to know the underlying reason that preceded the immobility. If you practice it, you will "resonate" with certain movements at certain moments in your life. The movements will just pop!

Every muscular action is a frequency, which when balanced is harmonious. But when imbalanced the compensatory pair creates a discord: One frequency compensates by being too dense and the other being compensated is too fine. They lack harmony. Like tightening the mast of a sailboat, if you tighten one wire too much, you overstretch the opposite wire. These small imbalances accumulate into a cacophony of noise that causes you aches and pain, and the cascade of emotions that accompanies it.

For example, there is a direct relationship between the piriformis muscle and the psoas muscle: When one is loose, the other is tight. When the psoas is too tight, you feel "doubled over" because you are constantly having to "lift everyone up or do everything yourself." The result is a loose piriformis. When the piriformis is too tight, you feel like you're always "playing catch-up" and "turning the wrong direction." The result is a loose psoas.

Conventional approaches would attempt to tighten the slackened, or "weak," muscles. An alternative used by ancient cultural folk wisdom from many countries is to bathe the tightness in mobility. A tight psoas could be addressed with pelvic circles in modified camel pose; whereas a tight piriformis could be addressed with hip circles in modified spinal

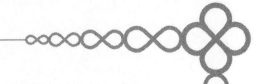

twisting pose. Each motion slowly shaves off the tension, one onion layer at a time.

In the early stages of reclaiming your bodily flow, you may be experiencing so much noise that you feel overwhelmed by where to start. Start anywhere; there are no "parts" to the body. The body may seem like a collection of different noises, but when you "tune in" you'll find that you have a choir singing; each voice you bring into tune makes the music that much more beautiful. My Intu-Flow system also allows you to tune up in a very systematic manner called the cephalocaudal-proximaldistal trend, the way your body most intuitively reclaims grace; hence the name Intu[itive] Flow®.

Conventional fitness approaches address imbalances by tightening the slack, the areas that are compensated. This belief derives from the pathological perspective that the body is broken and needs to be fixed with exercise. But you are not broken and do not need to be fixed. Tightening the slack is counterproductive because this just means that you're growing denser and more compressed, causing greater and stronger compensations, until the entire instrument, like overtightening violin strings, rips.

You are perfect *right now,* and I'll explain why. You can release the compensating tissues through mobility. You can discharge the stagnant, compressed areas through movement. But you can do so only by embracing the brilliance of your condition, by becoming thankful for your bodily intelligence.

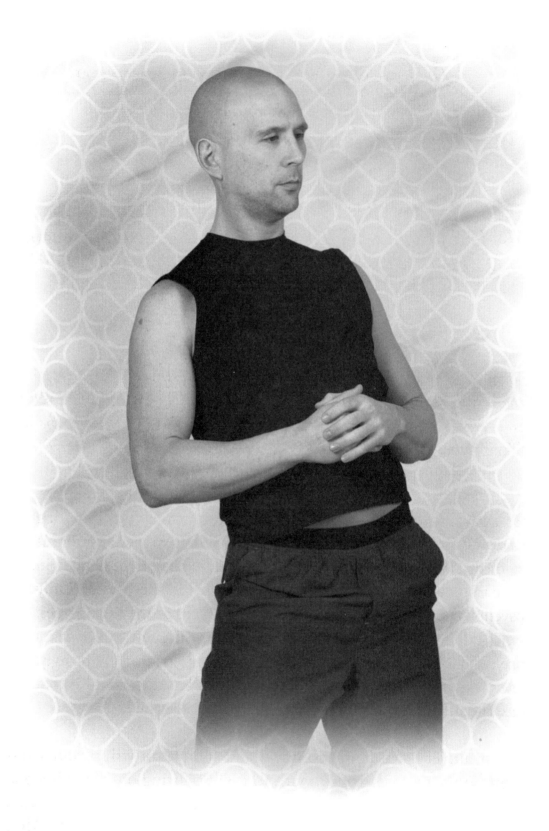

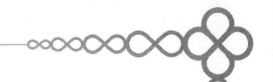

Mobility Expresses the Heart

"The love of our neighbor in all its fullness simply means being able to say to him, 'What are you going through?'"
Simone Weil

*T*he body speaks metaphorically, and the mind describes literally. When you feel like you've been sticking your neck out, you are. When you feel like you've been punched in the gut, kicked in the groin, slapped on the face, shouldering the responsibility, endlessly ribbed, like you have no footing, like someone is a pain in the neck, your body is reflecting it.

We are hardwired to communicate the truth. I've spent many years working with a dear colleague who has served as a body-language specialist for his government. When we review video, we analyze the physical ticks in response to particular comments and questions by the interviewer. Only the psychopaths communicate no truth alarms, for as the saying goes, neurotics build castles in the sky, but psychopaths live in them. It takes extensive deprogramming to be able to speak an untruth convincingly, and even then, it's only because the selected test failed to reveal it, not because the subject wasn't manifesting the truth somewhere.

Most anxiety causes you to fidget and squirm, to wring your hands with guilt, to cover your mouth to avoid blurting out the falsehood, to wipe your forehead with stress, to scratch your head in confusion as to the deception, to cross your arms to cover up the truth. All of

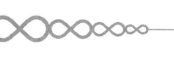

these ticks are fairly common, though anxiety can also be seen in the dilation of the pupils, the flicker in the rhythm of the heart, and the perspiration coming to the surface of the skin.

However, movement also communicates to us what we've been concealing from ourselves. What we fear facing, avoid confronting, and wish to deny. We cannot flee from an issue without running right into it. Unresolved trauma, and the fear-reactivity that results from it, is another example of emotions expressing themselves physically.

When I used to volunteer at a rape survivor clinic, many of the men and women held so much tension in their bodies that most movement caused physical pain. One wonderful woman named Rachel survived a rape by a man she had once been in a relationship with (at the time of the incident). Although she had been a professional dancer for 13 years, her entire posture had changed as a result of the attack and the violation of her trust. She had her "tail tucked between her legs," and her chest caved backward "with heartache."

She endured agony in her mid back and weakness in her knees. Her physician suggested an exercise program because she hadn't suffered any physical trauma, referring her to a personal trainer. The trainer advised squats to strengthen her weak thighs and cable pull-downs and rows to strengthen her shoulders to roll back. Rachel confided in me that she felt hopeless because these exercises only made her feel more pain, both physical and emotional.

Rachel and I discussed the violation she felt because the attacker was, at the time, her boyfriend. She said she felt "stabbed in the back and heartbroken" and upset that she had to flee her apartment without all of her belongings. Because we met at her dance studio, I asked Rachel if she would look in the mirror, and then I reflected back to her the description of her feelings she used.

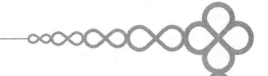

I discussed how delicately certain movements would need to be approached because they were both physical and emotional. For many rape survivors, feeling the stability and safety to stand tall as well as the courage to lift the heart takes time. We discussed the movements that she could practice, and how to create a safe place at her new home for practicing them.

I hadn't heard from Rachel in many years. Actually during the writing of this book, I received a surprise email from her. She admitted that the exercises were too emotional for her at first, so she ignored them and decided to return to her dance as therapy. She wrote about her difficulty with certain techniques and her inability to fully express herself with her dance, until she realized that the limitations she faced involved the very micromovements we had discussed in our session together.

Two years after our meeting, Rachel began practicing those movements. She explained that she felt the entire incident return to her in a flood of emotion, as if those movements were a tape recorder of the event. But she mustered the courage and practiced the movements safely in her home. She relied upon her close girlfriends and family to express how she had been feeling, and as a result she was able to distribute the charge of the experience throughout her support network.

Now Rachel feels confident in her "floor" with a sturdy "foundation." She shared with me how her dance now lets her "heart sing up to the heavens." She even said that she started to date again, a nurse by the name of John.

The amazing virtue of mobility is that we don't even need to know what the source issue is in order to receive 100% of its healing effects. Movement heals, just like music sooths, books inspire, and paintings awe, whether or not you understand why.

But you can also hasten the effect of healing movement, when you realize your inherent, perpetual perfection.

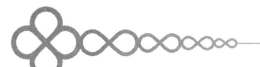

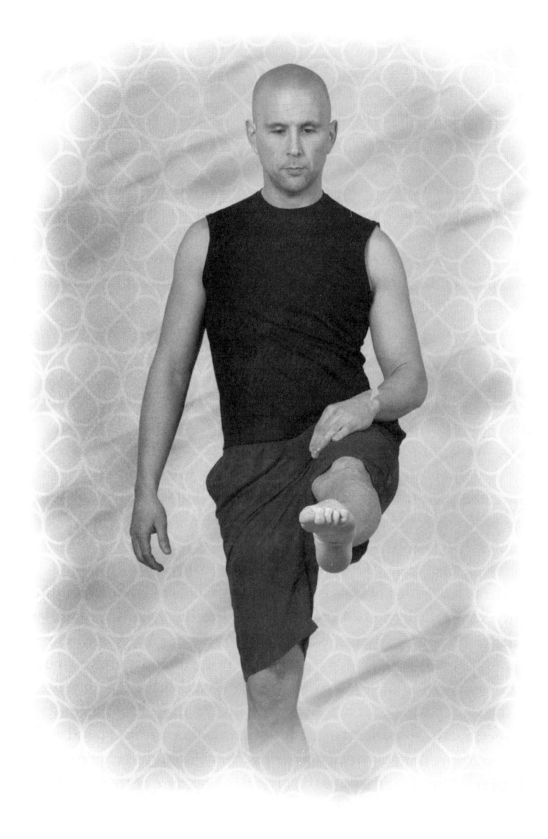

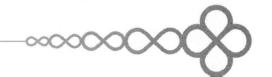

Owning Your Movement

One day, after several meetings with my international affiliates, Michael contacted me for a consultation. Michael was very upset because he had been experiencing extreme dissonance between his religious life and his physical life. Coming from an orthodox faith, and a family history of obesity, he expressed his disconnection with his physical body over the years.

His story isn't unique, unfortunately. Most of us know the kind of disconnect Michael's talking about, where we don't feel plugged into who we are in our physical life because we start to believe that our physical body is just a broken vessel that we will eventually dispose of. I know I felt this coming from a family whose traditional background was Seventh-Day Adventist; my mother wasn't allowed to dance or sing outside church functions.

Michael and I engaged in a private consultation where we went through my Sonnon Method of discussing the specific areas of discomfort he had been feeling in his movement, the areas that made him most self-conscious. These are the areas that restrict us most and congest our energy, making us feel bloated, stagnant, and thick.

By targeting these particular areas, Michael then started to reveal how there are certain movements such as sprawls and hula hoops that made him feel most embarrassed, particularly because of their implied sexuality. This is not unusual for most men, and it can be the same for women as well.

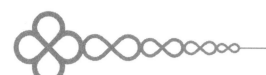

I asked Michael to name the advantages that his orthodoxy background brought to his physical life, and he looked at me as if I were crazy. "There aren't any," he first replied. But through a process I've learned from Dr. John Demartini, I kept on him. Michael made his first point on how his faith allowed him to not be egotistical about his physicality, to not be fixated on his appearance, to not place an overemphasis on his physique. This allowed him to concentrate on his health.

The list of advantages grew longer and longer as Michael expanded on how his physical life became crucial for him to be of greater service in his religious community and gave him greater stamina for ceremonies, greater mental acuity for studying his texts, greater relaxation so that he would not be disturbed by aches and pains, and increased energy so that he could be more enthusiastic and motivational in his presentations to his gatherings. And I could see the transformation happening as Michael scribbled out one bullet point after another. When he filled a second page, he stopped and looked up with a grin, saying, *"I had no idea."*

We returned to the individual movements, and with a smirk on his face, Michael started to "own his movement." We designed a program for him that would concentrate on these areas — mobility, yoga, and athletic conditioning — all three wings of CST. But slapping a large hand on my back and gesturing to his body, Michael said, "I have to thank you, Scott. I knew that your private consultations were a big investment, but I felt like I didn't have anywhere else to turn. I was skeptical because I never thought that I would be able to see the bridge between my religious life and my physical one. But now I *do* feel like I own my movement."

Breakthrough moments such as Michael's really make my vocation such a privilege. Michael embodied his beliefs, and in all of the years of success I've seen prosper with my Method, I expect that he will continue to feel greater ownership of his movement as his practice deepens.

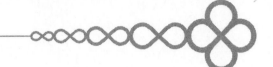

We can each learn from Michael's leadership. If we embrace our movement — the familial, social, financial, vocational, mental, and spiritual — each of the other aspects of our life will develop simultaneously and synergistically.

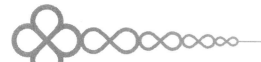

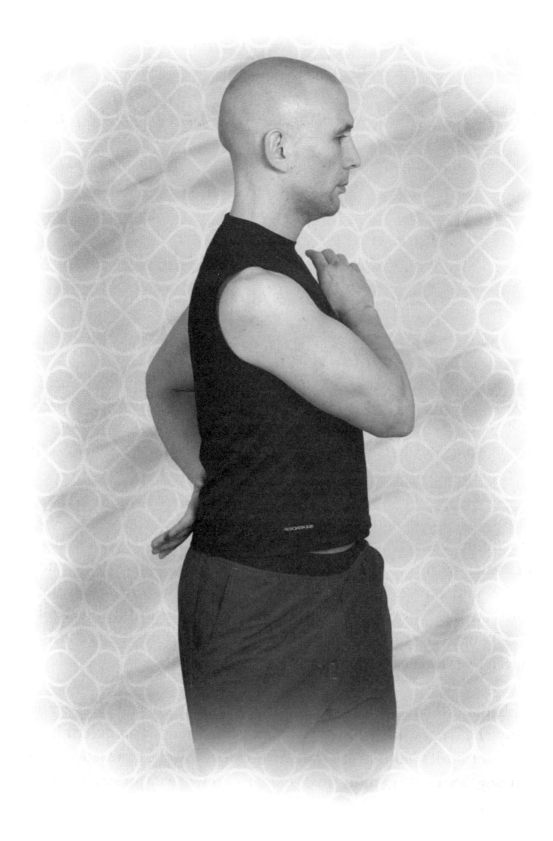

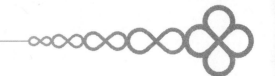

Loving Your Immobility XVII

*"Whatever you feel uncomfortable about,
and don't love, is stopping you."*
Dr. John Demartini

You can regain balance, or re-harmonize, by Following Lovingly Ordered Wisdom. Your body expresses what you're neglecting to pay attention to. It perfectly manifests precisely what it needs to communicate; the more you ignore its requests, the more obstreperous it becomes as it tries to regain your love, support, and attention.

Conventional health approaches aren't healthy at all. They don't regard health improvement, but focus on "fixing disease." This perspective views issues within the body as pathologies. But to allow flow into your life, and express it physically, reframe what you're experiencing within you as a positive. This isn't idealistic optimism but practical reality. Whatever obstacle we're stumbling over is something within we haven't yet learned how to love.

I had a difficult childhood, harder than some but not all. Because of my challenges, I learned to rely upon persistence and determination. An authority telling me that my "defects" would prevent me from doing something motivated me to "find a way or make one," as Hannibal said.

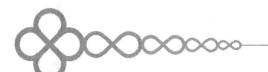

Somewhere along my growth, that coping skill started to operate unchecked. Whenever I saw anything that looked beyond my abilities, I feverishly threw myself into it until I could do it. I didn't do this intelligently though, and would often pursue multiple extremely challenging tasks simultaneously. One day I set several personal records in different physical disciplines. I awoke the next day with about 20% strength in my left arm and severe pain in my neck. I could barely press myself off the ground in a push-up without falling face-first.

Calling upon my health care team, I received treatment from three chiropractors, two physical therapists, two kinesiologists, and a massage therapist. Each gave some relief, but no "cure" resulted. However, I was able to identify the specific muscle, my levator scapuli, as the compensating culprit. Mobility restored me to approximately 85% of my natural strength, but complete relief eluded me. I met with a Reiki master in Australia who pointed out that it was the one area I couldn't "reach" with my hands. Years of mobility training have allowed me to know the attachment points and to persuade muscular tension to release by touch. But I couldn't get to this issue.

The Reiki master indicated that I should consider the fact that I deliberately created an issue I couldn't "get my hands on." With a twinkle in her eye she shoved me, because someone of my experience would not realize the intentionality behind such a genius safety valve. If I couldn't reach the area to heal it, then I would be forced to stop. Once I was compelled to sit still, all of my concurrent overtraining and competitiveness came into full clarity.

I manifested this wonderful control mechanism to govern my own ability to injure myself. Whenever I approached injuring myself, or burning out, I would turn off this muscle and as a result become incapable of continuing potentially dangerous levels of activity. What an amazing blessing!

As a very pragmatic person who requires empirical evidence to accept most things, I am not prone to believe in the placebo effect. This idea, however, made complete sense to me, and I accepted it at face value. I blessed my intelligently designed safety valve, practiced my yoga on the beach that morning, and then let it go. The next day, the soreness throughout my upper back caused me to chuckle, as it felt as if I had just left the Rolfing table. Any bound flow just decided to release overnight. I returned to full strength in just 24 hours.

I feel thankful, however, that I still have that safety valve in place. Even though the Reiki master prepared me with some energetic techniques to normalize the sudden whoosh I still feel when I encounter something that I cannot yet do, or worse, when someone challenges me by claiming I am incapable of some task, I still need that help. And those techniques still weave their magic, preventing me from diving into the nearest breach.

When you face an issue, ask yourself, In what way is it protecting you? How is the issue you're experiencing of benefit to you? I learned from Dr. John Demartini that sitting down and writing an advantages and disadvantages list for each issue allows you to see objectively what it is that you have not yet learned to love.

Once you realize that a particular issue is protecting you from harm, you learn to love it. Take, for example, a herniated disc. The tendency to stretch the neck chin to chest releases the tight muscles, but it causes the disc to "squirt" out even more. The tightness acts as a temporary splint until you can experience recovery in the bulging disc. Specific mobility exercises will help you do that, once you stop fighting the issue and start loving it for its protective nature.

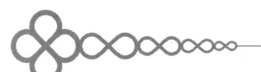
NEEDING NO HANDOUT

I'd like to share one last truly inspirational story with you. For many years I taught martial arts. Some students were world champions, but one man in particular honored me with the highlight of my coaching career.

Joseph was born without arms or legs. He had stumps that allowed him to manipulate objects, but he accepted anything but immobility. When Joseph began training with me, he was already a black belt in one style of martial art, a beautiful artist whose drawings would take your breath away.

He never complained, and he always found humor in what he joked were his "shortcomings." Every camp that he participated in found each participant training harder, laughing often, and developing more than he or she would have without the gift of Joseph's enlightening presence.

Obviously, Joseph and I had to modify each exercise to meet his needs. But he equally had a learning advantage because he didn't have to learn how to not think with his hands and feet, which most people do. Most of our cerebral matter is dedicated to our hands and feet, and with those absent from Joseph, all of that brain power went to the interior joints of the hips, shoulders, and spine. His sensitivity dazzled everyone.

At one of my camps, Joseph and his partner were having difficulties with a particular drill. I unwittingly asked, "Can I give you a hand?" The words escaped my mouth before I realized what I had said. Joseph replied, "I'll take two, Scott!" This remark left all of us in stitches from laughter. Joseph would ask for help, but he never once begrudged his condition. He learned at an incredible rate, because he couldn't afford to have ego in the way of his mobility.

Joseph and I met for dinner one evening and discussed his condition. At one point he leaned forward and extended his arm toward me to shake. As I clasped his arm and shook it with my hand, he smiled and said some of the most indelibly etched words in my memory: "Scott, thanks for not coddling me. Even though the modifications we created were necessary, you never patronized me. I'm just as mobile as everyone else. I just have less to do. So thanks for creating drills which could challenge me."

Joseph "got it." He felt blessed by his situation because it allowed him to experience the world with integrity. He couldn't pretend to perform the exercises and fake his way through training. In each drill, he earned it through sweat and blood. Where others fully "capable" would complain about the challenges and whine about the hardships, Joseph treasured them. Although Joseph honored me by allowing me to teach him, I feel as if I learned so much more from his presence in my life.

Mobility is a state of mind. It's how we consciously interact and perceive the world to be. We can view life as a prison or a playground, and the choice is our own to make. There is a path to opening the prison door and returning to the playground of life. It can be done through movement.

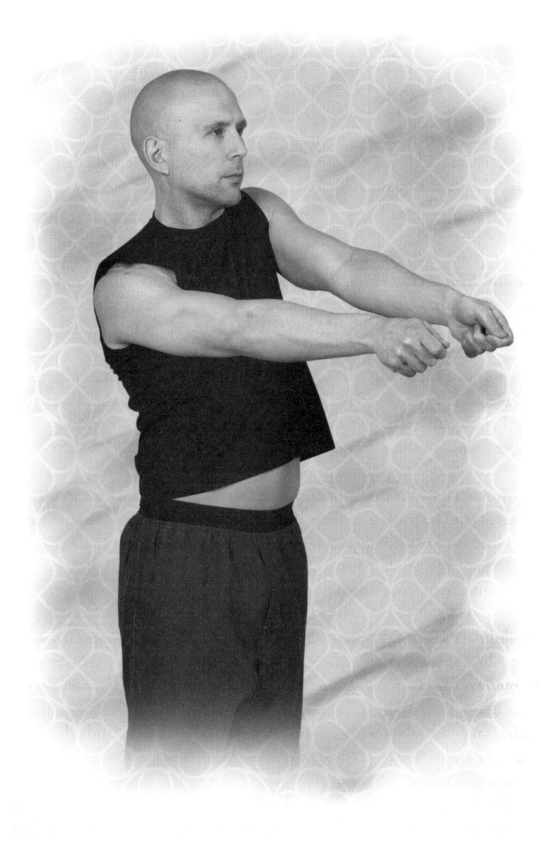

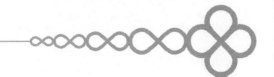

The Problem with Stretching XVIII

We have all been told to stretch out our muscles before and after exercising. This suggestion, however, is based on what a small percentage of the population can handle without injury. Most people find little benefit from this stretching myth.

When you stretch you take a muscle and force it to lengthen until it changes shape and stays longer. Think of taking a rubber band, lengthening it, tacking it down, and, over time, watching how the rubber band loses its elasticity and adopts the new length.

Your joints need elasticity in order to protect themselves, to keep everything packed tightly. Dancers, gymnasts, and contortionists — the most flexible people in the world — suffer debilitating injuries in later life due to permanent changes in tissue length. The lax, loose connective tissue doesn't protect them from injury.

Flexibility measures the increased range of motion due to an improved strength/surrender ratio. You never "use" flexibility in real life because it's merely a measurement, just like the direct distance between two cities doesn't help you travel along the winding roads, the congested traffic, and the delays with stoplights, construction work, and adverse weather conditions.

Flexibility is like using the bench press (which is where the term *benchmark* originated for determining fitness) as a measure of one's

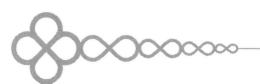

ability to function in daily life. Think of your scale at home. How much you weigh has no direct relationship to how healthy and fit you are. As a matter of fact, as you become fitter, you'll gain muscle, and weigh more! The same is true of your joints. As you become healthier in lax joints, your joints will become tighter, and as a result safer, more reliable, and stronger.

DEBUNKING THE STRETCHING MYTH

When you're given the opportunity, knowledge, and experience to question whether stretching is health and longevity virtue, you'll discover that stretching is not a high-premium activity. Due to my genetic challenges, stretching wasn't an option, so luckily, I sought out the world's best authorities on the topic and absorbed the wisdom of their research.

Here are some of the main insights of the best of the best around the world, from the men and women who have pioneered the fields of biomechanics and biotensegrity:

- Flexibility is **not** a primary characteristic of health and performance.
- Flexibility is **not** a form of injury prevention.
- Injury does **not** result from insufficient stretching.
- Injury does **not** necessarily mean that the tissue was maximally stretched.
- Static stretching is **not** safe and productive.
- Dynamic stretching (mobility drills) is **not** unsafe and unproductive.
- Daily stretching is **not** mandatory for flexibility maintenance.
- Flexibility is **not** last to arrive and first to go. (Pain is.)
- Flexibility does **not** require deforming the tissue length.

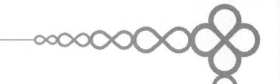

DOES IT STRETCH BACK!?

Flexibility measures specific direction. Static stretching suggests that to increase the flexibility, one needs to pull the tissue in an isolated range of motion until the stress causes permanent deformation, and the tissue becomes incapable of returning to its original state. But deforming your tissue creates a high risk of hazards for mobile security and joint health.

> Conventional thought assumes that stretching after activity can prevent the muscle from healing at a shorter length. However, even if the stretching were to prevent shortening, connective tissue will stiffen regardless due to the process of healing and aging.

Over the years of any activity (even sitting on the couch), you cause microtrauma to your connective tissue. You heal, but only when scar tissue forms. The scar mends the wound by pulling and shortening the tissue. From stretching, you endure an irreversible process of increasing collagen (scar tissue) and decreasing elastin (your elasticity).

> Elasticity is the ability to return to the original state following deformation. To increase the elasticity of a tissue, you apply positive stress (not strain) through a range of motion. You remove the stress after the initial stiffness stops but before the tissue permanently deforms so the tissue returns to its original state. This stress increases the capacity for storage of "elastic energy."

RUBBER BAND MAN

The ability to generate stored elastic energy (SEE) relates to the strength of the tissue, or its "tensile strength" — the maximum stress you can withstand before you break. Your "ductility" (how malleable you are) decreases as you get closer to your breaking point. On the other end of the spectrum, your elasticity increases as you get closer to your breaking point. Like pulling the string of a bow, the farther you pull back the string, the harder it becomes to pull. But the farther the arrow will fly.

My teachers called this concept "viscosity" — the degree to which an object stays at rest when acted upon by an outside force. Your body constricts, congeals, and thickens when acted upon by stresses from within and without. Like stirring a bowl of honey, your viscosity is your resistance to force; the greater the viscosity, the greater the force and time required to cause deformation.

To understand this concept, pull a rubber band in two opposite directions. The farther you pull, the harder you must pull. Pull the rubber band one inch, it gains 5 units of elastic energy. Pull a second inch, and it produces 10 additional units of elastic energy (15 total). Pull a third inch, and you produce 20 more units (35 total). As you continue to pull the rubber band, the force grows exponentially.

This means that you adapt to both the intensity and the duration of stress, and two things can occur: In the rubber band example, too much stress can cause the rubber band to snap, or the rubber band can begin to deform permanently. Unfortunately, conventional static stretching causes one or both of these health risks. Let's talk about the "snap"!

THE STRETCH REFLEX

All of us have slipped on ice at some point in our lives. As you slip on the ice, your body goes off balance. Reflexively, you try to "right yourself" to regain your equilibrium. So what's going on inside you physiologically during this involuntary event to keep from falling? The tissue stretched when you slipped — say your hamstring or groin — contracts to the original position fast and hard. Suddenly you tear, due to the stretch reflex: A muscle stretched by an external force too far or too fast contracts to oppose the stretch even at its own expense.

Tissue does *not* have to be maximally stretched to be torn. Tears result from a combination of sudden stretch and muscular contraction.

Let's return to our rubber band. Imagine the rubber band has a maximum of 50 units of elastic potential. You pulled it three inches and produced 35 units of elastic energy. If you pull the rubber band one final inch, you will produce 40 more units of elastic energy for a total of 75. But because this exceeds the tensile strength of the rubber band, the rubber band ruptures during the pull (when you hit 50 total units, its maximum strength). Static stretching is like this, and the type of dangerous flexibility it produces makes tearing connective tissue or rupturing a joint much more likely.

Some misunderstand this to mean that injuries occur when a muscle is stretched beyond its limit. As a result they wrongly assume that you prevent injuries by elongating the muscles of the connective tissues. But this is like thinking that you can stop drunk-driving accidents by making the roads wider.

Tears do not happen because tissues have been maximally lengthened but due to the special combination of sudden stretch and contraction called the stretch reflex.

FLEXIBILITY IS SPEED SPECIFIC

If you slowly pull the rubber band and hold it at a certain length, it will begin to deform permanently, and lose its elasticity. My teachers called this "viscoelasticity" — the combination of viscosity and elasticity. What this basically means is that your tissue adapts to not only the distance you pull it, but also how long you pull it. The longer you stretch, even with the same intensity, the more the tissue will start to permanently deform.

Heat also affects this process. Long-distance stretches for long duration under high temperature cause permanent changes in tissue length. Remember, that's not necessarily healthy because these deformations may seem like you're becoming more flexible, but you're really exposing yourself to harm. Just because under high heat, for long duration, at a

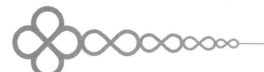

low intensity you have a measure of flexibility doesn't mean that when you're not hot and you suddenly have a high-intensity contraction (like when you slip on the ice) you'll have the flexibility. It's speed specific.

When your body needs to recover, stabilize, or function, it contracts. And if you haven't developed the range of motion with real-world speed, you will tear. You can't increase your mobility — your essential coordination — through static stretches.

Your stretch reflex engages whenever a muscle is stretched suddenly or dramatically, or both. The muscle spindles — the two special receptors — that control the stretch reflex are sensitive to stretch magnitude and to speed. Static stretch may or may not reset the first receptor, but it is completely ineffective for the latter. As a result, flexibility is speed specific.

PLASTIC CHANGES

Some tissues are less injury prone when stressed rapidly. For instance, ligaments are composed of wavy collagen fibers. Uncoiled, the fibers become susceptible to injury. If taken too far, a ligament tears. Slow loading causes uncoiling through taking the slack out of the fibers; quick loading does not allow sufficient time for a ligament to recover.

Cartilage is equally less injury prone when quickly loaded. Cartilage decreases the stress in a joint by decreasing the friction between bones and by distributing the load over the surface of the joint. Cartilage is composed of 20–40% collagen and 60–80% water, and as a result it behaves like a sponge. When compressed, it decreases the protection between bones. However, with rapid loading the fluid does not have sufficient time to be squeezed out and it can better absorb shock.

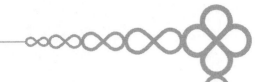

HEALTH RISKS OF STATIC STRETCHING

The practice of increasing flexibility through static stretching is a serious health danger. With wear and tear, the collagen/elastin ratio changes in favor of collagen. So as we grow older, with decreased elasticity, connective tissue becomes more likely to snap.

> In our youth, dropping into a straddle split seemed like a desirable ability, but it has nothing to do with health, and even less to do with longevity. As you grow older, you discover that it's not how far you can stretch that's important but how gracefully you can recover from any sudden changes. That gracefulness is also the essence of physical mastery in all sports.

As a result, we must become flexible in dynamic motion at the speed of life.

SHORT-RANGE STIFFNESS

Most people tend to feel better after they've gone through a stretching routine. They are likely to feel loose and more relaxed. This is healthy but should be properly understood. Physiologically, when inactive we experience short-range stiffness. After surpassing this initial resistance, we feel a substantial reduction in the stiffness. This is a temporary, not permanent. Concentrate on overcoming the stiffness, but don't exceed it or hold it for a long duration.

THE ESSENCE OF SYNERGY: RANGE OF MOTION

Range of motion, or the ability to move through, about, and around a joint's full potential, applies directly to daily life. My teachers in biomechanics called this "essential synergy" to represent the idea that the whole of a joint's movement cannot reasonably be quantified. Just like you can't measure the infinity in basic mathematics, your mobility is both a quantity and quality of life.

Soviet scientist and physician Alexander Bogomoletz said wisely, "Man is as old as his connective tissues." The corollary to this statement is expressed in the title to Editha Hearn's 1967 book *You Are as Young as Your Spine.* Basically, if we rely on tissue elasticity for flexibility, we'll lose it. Your coordination determines your age.

Range of motion can be used to describe the mobility remaining in a joint. For example, if a cyclist rides 100 miles or more per week but doesn't move his or her hips through their full range regularly, he or she might experience limited mobility at the hip joint. The term *range of motion* could be used to refer to this measurement of the mobility remaining after limitation.

Have you ever sat at the computer all day? Doing so probably made the front of your shoulders tighten and overstretched muscles in the upper back and neck. This imbalance in muscle tone limits the range of motion of the shoulder. Although most people feel apt to rub their painful necks, standing and performing overhead shoulder circles will help much more quickly and fully.

Range of motion is expressed in degrees of joint angle or circumference (depending upon what type of joint is being measured). Each joint has an established normal range, based on what that joint does and where the two bones that compose it can move no more. In other words, the normal range of movement is determined by the architecture of the bones and the soft tissues that surround the joint to hold it together. Range of motion is very related to flexibility.

MOBILITY PRACTICE
Mobility practice is more important for not only athletic performance but also anti-aging. Mobility can be used for an energetic supercharge as well as a warm-up for more strenuous activities. You can also use mobility practice for active recovery when you don't want to train strenuously.

Unlike static stretching, mobility means movement (not position) into the full natural range of motion of each joint through voluntary control. Unlike static stretching, in mobility practice don't try to hold an extreme position. Pass through it slowly and smoothly without forcing the tissues to deform, and by allowing the muscles to relax voluntarily.

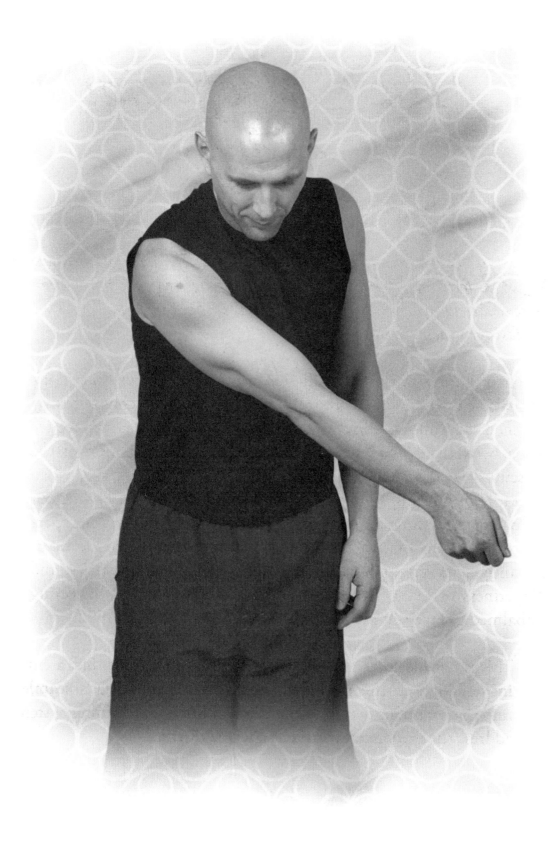

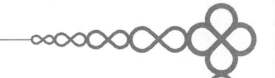

The Myofascial Matrix

Although for the past several decades bodybuilding has reduced the focus of athleticism to a theory of isolated muscular action, the musculoskeletal system is an irreducible matrix. Even one small stressor in the myofascia impacts the entire matrix.

Sheets of fibrous myofascial adhesion can form anywhere and block normal, healthy function. Too often, fascia has been considered by the medical world as merely packing material, simply a connective tissue between areas of function. The contemporary notion of the musculoskeletal system developed only about 250 years ago, when the knife in hunting and the scalpel in dissection served to "cut out the parts" of the human organism. Unfortunately, what was cut apart and what drained out are the very animating structure that lends us the antigravitational potential we have. The mobility, elasticity, and slipperiness of living fascia can never be appreciated by dissecting embalmed cadavers in medical school. (Leahy and Mock, 1992.)

This is not meant as an exhaustive overview, but rather just a cursory introduction to the myofascial matrix. This intro leads seamlessly into the conscious design of the Circular Strength Training System to address the myofascial matrix as a whole matrix.

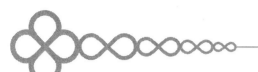

SNAGS IN THE SWEATER

Myofascia has an appearance similar to a very densely woven spider's web or wool sweater, and lines and covers nearly everything in the body. It surrounds every muscle bone, nerve, artery, and vein as well as all of our internal organs, including the heart, lungs, brain, and spinal cord. The most interesting aspect about the myofascial matrix is that it is actually one single fascial sheath that essentially has pockets, one for each structure. In other words, we are one muscle with hundreds of insertion points. Every aspect of the body is interwoven with every other, like yarn in a sweater.

Myofascia is a connective tissue that forms a three-dimensional web surrounding and supporting the muscular, skeletal, and visceral (organs) components of the body. Fascial restrictions bind down and exert pressure and stress on the body and its soft tissue structures, causing pain and dysfunction. Like a pull in the yarn of a sweater, fascial restrictions can affect your whole body. For athletics, this leads to severe and systemwide "leaking" of power, potential, and practice.

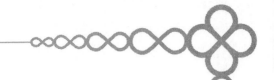

The Fascial Layers

*T**he following is a cursory look at some of the forms that fascia takes.*

Superficial fascia is attached to the underside of your skin. Capillary channels and lymph vessels run through this layer, and so do many nerves. Subcutaneous fat is attached to it. In healthy superficial fascia, skin moves fluidly over the surface of muscles. In most people, especially athletes due to bodybuilding, it is often stuck. In the superficial fascia, there is a great potential to store excess fluid and metabolites, which are the breakdown products of informational substances and other chemicals in your body.

Deep fascia is much tougher and denser material that separates large sections of the body, such as the abdominal cavity. Deep fascia covers some areas like huge sheets to protect them and shape them. Deep fascia also separates muscles and organs. The bag-like covering around the heart (the pericardium), the lining of the chest cavity (the pleura), and the area between external genitals and anus (the perineum) are all made up of specialized deep fascia.

Subserous fascia is the loose tissue that covers internal organs and holds the rich network of blood and lymph vessels that keeps them moist. Even cells have a type of cytoskeleton connected to the fascia network, which is what gives cells shape and allows them to function.

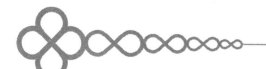

The dural tube surrounds and protects the spinal cord and contains the cerebrospinal fluid. This tube connects to the membranes surrounding your brain. Together, they hold and protect the craniosacral system.

Fascia is also the material that forms adhesions and scar tissue. When healthy, ground substance has a gelatinous consistency (like gelfoam medical packing, or like sprayed-on Styrofoam insulation) so that it can absorb the forces that are created during movement, contraction, or trauma. It can change from liquid to gel to solid form — hardening and losing elasticity and becoming like a glue or cement poured into fascial gaps, which tightens myofascia. It cannot reverse this state and return to liquid form without intervention (e.g., tactical manipulation, mobility drills, and decompression exercise such as yoga).

The ground substance transfers nutrients from where they break down into usable materials to where they will be used and removes waste products from these areas of use. This exchange and transport through diffusion takes part in the ground substance. Without it the tissue starves and becomes brittle and toxic.

Another important job for your ground substance is to maintain the distance between connective tissue fibers. This prevents adhesions from forming, and keeps tissue supple and elastic. When critical distance is not maintained, fibers become cross-linked by newly synthesized collagen, which is also part of the fascia. Collagen cross-links are arranged haphazardly, unlike healthy linkages, and are hard to break up.

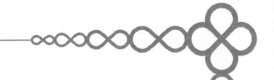

Biotensegrity XXI

Various manifestations of residual tension, sensory motor amnesia, fear-reactivity, and myofascial density usually result from compensatory tension created as a reaction to a source injury; hence our adherence to the maxim "the site is not the source."

After the acute phase of the injury, our nervous system adapts to the background "noise" of the issue. At the end of the acute phase there are no longer any symptoms of the source issue. But as soon as the source stops manifesting symptoms, elsewhere in the body sites of symptoms may begin to erupt. And the chase begins.

> Mobility addresses the source issues of tension in the myofascial matrix: our spidery ubiquity of connective tissue and electric goo, which we call muscle. By chasing issues (through particular exercise selection and sequence) to the source, we release the sites from the ongoing compensatory strain while eventually liberating the source tension to allow it to heal through the body's natural healing process. It's how we, in concert with the aid of our health care team, "get out of our own way" of healing. As a result, yoga can produce immediate if not eventual global reorganization, cheering the body into its innate pain-free carriage.

Buckminster Fuller and Dr. Stephen Levin's biotensegrity model offers a clear underlying structure of organic tissue. The biotensegrity

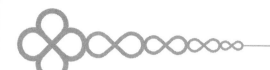

model explains the nebulous interdependence of the body's structural components. It goes far beyond the conventional model of muscle-tendon-ligament reaction to injury by including the entire structure of the organism as a potential home for referred dysfunction.

> "The word 'tensegrity' is an invention: a contraction of 'tensional integrity.' Tensegrity describes a structural-relationship principle in which structural shape is guaranteed by the finitely closed, comprehensively continuous, tensional behaviors of the system and not by the discontinuous and exclusively local compression member behaviors. Tensegrity provides the ability to yield increasingly without ultimately breaking or coming asunder." (Fuller, Buckminster. *Synergetics,* MacMillan, New York, 1975.)

In an incredibly instructionally dense DVD on his biotensegrity work, Dr. Levin explains that bodily tissues involve interwoven tension icosahedra. These complex triangular trusses balance stability and mobility by creating a myofascial sea of continuous tension pulling inward while the compressive struts of the hard bones push outward.

> Biotensegrity serves to provide explanations that remain elusive to observers viewing bodily phenomena through the lens of the Newtonian mechanical model of human structure. An understanding of the biotensegrity model allows great clarification of the ways in which the body's gravitational support system responds to stress, strain, trauma, and fear.

Simply stated, when the tissues become overwhelmed by stress (mechanical, physiological, or emotional/biochemical), they lose their resilient ability to adapt and compensate. As a result, the myofascial matrix responds by altering the stored tension and elastic potential of the tissues, pulling in one place and creating a strain somewhere down the track. Our normal, neutral, and responsive bodily structure mutates into a highly strained, linearly stiffened, highly charged form. This latter transformation explains how the slightest poor form, meager stress, or emotional arousal can result in instant and even acute injury anywhere along the bound chains of tension.

Unfortunately, most people live in this pre-tense state, and over time adapt to it — or worse, progress upon it — like with any conditioning. The unknowing, innocent public is bombarded by exercise gurus and companies that advise high-tension breath holding, which not only reinforces this pre-tense condition but also can make it snap anywhere along the tension chain!

If we experience pain, tightness, weakness, and so on, we can assume we have a movement problem, which can often be detected via the process of mobilizing an area and thereby discovering uncomfortable tension and breath holding. Regardless of whether the problem at hand is a site symptom or the source issue, the structural dysfunction can be addressed through movement and breath work, employed to re-educate the body to move without pain, and exhaling through the discomfort. This is the role of individual asana as a personal diagnostic.

All movement expresses at the joints. With only a few exceptions, if we move, we move the joints. So if we have a global movement problem, we must by definition have a local movement problem. Before one can address the disintegration (global movement problems), one must address the local movement problems.

How do we address local movement problems? We must recover the local movement quality. We move the joint while the rest of the body remains in a neutral, static position. A helpful metaphor is replacing a broken cog in a machine. As soon as the teeth of the new cog sync up with the others (breath, movement, and structure integrating), then the machine instantly runs well again.

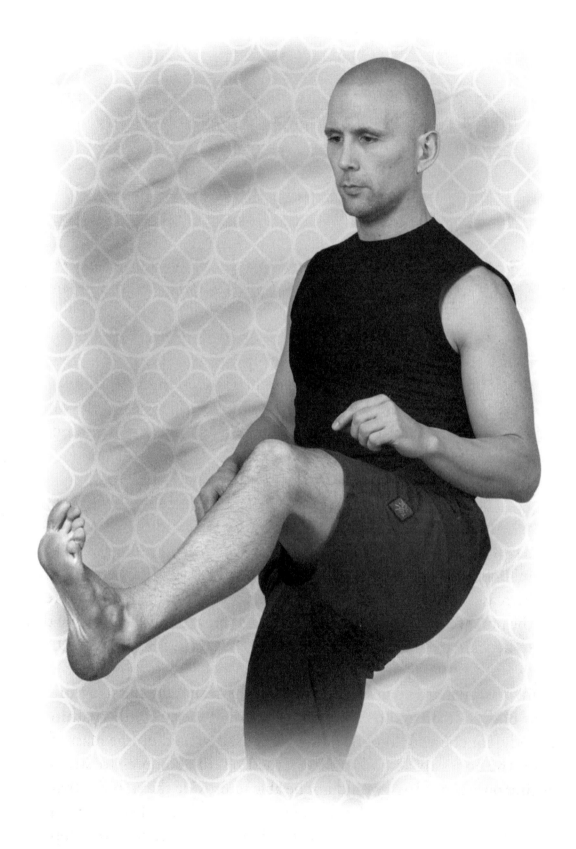

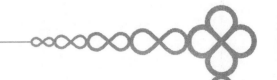

The "Double Bag"

Mobility impacts the "double-bag system" of the musculoskeletal system. Myofascia (muscle/fascia) is fascia that is related to musculoskeletal tissue.

The "inner bag" that cling wraps like cellophane is called periosteum, and where it holds two or more bones together is called the joint capsule. The hard substances within (bone and cartilage) are cushioned by synovial fluid within the capsule, and bathed when healthy by ground substance throughout.

> The "outer bag" is called fascial tissue and contains an electric goo called muscle tissue. Where the outer bag is tacked down to the inner bag is called the attachment or insertion point. The cellular membranes in these attachment areas can become extremely convoluted, which increases the surface area and changes the angle of force. This increases the potential for things to get stuck together, and causes the tissue there to become more easily torn. (Simons, Travell, and Simons, 1999.)

The myofascial matrix plays an essential role in the support and structure of our bodies. It surrounds and attaches to all of the structures within the body, functioning like the guide wires used to hold up the mast of a ship. The bones are actually passive structures, like compressive struts pushing outwards. They would not be able to provide the stability that they do without the sea of continuous tension that is being pulled back inward by the fascia net. Think of bones as the mast of the ship

and the fascia as the guide wires that maintain the appropriate degree of tension that allows the body to remain upright with the proper equilibrium, to propel itself through various physical tasks within the six degrees of freedom, and to withstand the buffeting of forces it experiences within the gravitational field and when in collision with other objects and subjects.

This delicate balance was named biotensegrity by Dr. Steven Levin, and relates to the engineering concept of tensegrity developed by Buckminster Fuller. Dr. Levin explains how the compressive struts push outward while floating in a sea of continuous tension pulling inward for optimal balance and propulsion through the field of gravity.

ADAPTATION AND RESTRICTION

A healthy myofascial web remains relaxed and wavy with the ability to stretch like a rubber band, moving fluidly without restriction and returning back to its original shape when the muscular action diminishes.

When we experience physical trauma, myofascia loses pliability. It becomes tight, restricted, and a source of tension to the rest of the body, like a constant snag in a sweater or an overly tight guide wire on the mast of a ship threatening to snap the mast should another adverse wind suddenly fill the sails.

This adaptation from collision, surgery, or habitual poor form/structure has a cumulative effect over time on the skeletal structure. These effects begin during infancy and progress throughout life with trauma, but also with all stresses placed upon our highly adaptive organism.

Unbalanced, unresolved, or unregulated adaptation negatively impacts flexibility, agility, coordination, strength, power, and stamina. To return to the metaphor of the snagged sweater or the overtaut mast wires, myofascial adaptation is a determining factor in the ability to

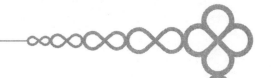

withstand stress and strain during strenuous activity, such as athletics, as well as during normal everyday activities.

To understand how the myofascial matrix may impact a seemingly unrelated part of our body, imagine the fascia as a wool sweater. If you were to attach a hook to the sweater at the hip and pull in a downward direction away from the body, you would feel the effect of the pull at the opposite shoulder.

OVERCOMPENSATION

An imbalanced matrix means that some muscles pull too tightly while others are too loose. These chains of tension form snags in the sweater we call compensations. In a compensation pattern, one or more myofascial bands remain in an inhibited state and need continuous assistance from other myofascial bands in order for the body to continue functioning. These chains of tension, called residual tension chains, run the length of the body.

> Myofascial bands define structures of contiguous tissue that perform a related action or maintain structural integrity along one side of an entire limb, or even along the entire body. Within these structures are many separate, unique muscle bellies. Thus, myofascial bands cross multiple joints in performing their function, named "anatomy trains" by Thomas Myers in his book of the same name.

Myofascial bands coalesce primarily into a longitudinal axis along one side of a limb or along the entire body. This is where we find the "grain" of the related muscles all running in one general direction. Therefore, while the fascia weaves itself through a muscle belly, it continues on as an insertion tendon, then blends itself into the periosteum and joint capsule ligaments. Nearby, one or more origin tendons arise, and the fascia extends into the next one down the line.

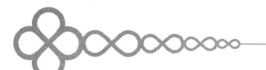

One myofascial band compensates for one or more others because the motor center thinks it is the best one for the job. The motor center knows, via proprioceptive feedback, that others are not working efficiently. The motor center also knows that some are always there, working every time it requires them for a task.

If you were the boss of some workers who were lazy and others who were completely dependable and you absolutely had to get a project done immediately, whom would you call upon to do it? Neurologically, the answer is based upon the principle of facilitation: The most active, dependable muscles will be recruited first when compensation is required.

Myofascial chains may be weak (compensated) and/or tight (compensating) and they are highly injury prone. A tight band is compensating for other weak or loose bands. Whereas a strong band can handle the stress of tension internal or external, a weak band is unable to do so. The muscle, already compromised by compensation, is unable to rise to the challenge. Eventually, it will either tear in the belly or, most likely, begin to fray at the insertion point.

Compensation should not be viewed as pathology. It is an evolutionarily stable survival mechanism, without which we would fall down every time we took one step with a weak psoas, for example. Without compensation, every trauma to the musculoskeletal system could be debilitating. Presumably, our ancestors would have been unable to get away from a saber-toothed tiger just because of weakness in a couple of leg muscles. The myofascial matrix recruits whatever it needs to accomplish the task set forth by the central nervous system.

However, without resolving the compensation, the tension chains then progress, like all adaptation, to internal muscular resistance.

Over time, myofascia hardens into thick, leathery straps in order to maintain the imbalanced structure called myofascial density. The hardening leads to loss of neuromuscular firing potential, and as a result the brain can no longer send the request for movement. This condition was named sensory motor amnesia by Thomas Hanna in his book *Somatics: Reawakening the Mind's Control of Movement, Flexibility, and Health.* When moved into an inhibited, restricted, or amnesic range of motion, the myofascial matrix then defensively braces with spasm called fear-reactivity.

Once the motor center begins using it for one compensation pattern, it is more likely to go to it in future situations that require compensation. Through your mobility practice, Circular Strength Training locates these tight bands and reprograms their motor function to delete this tension from the motor programs so that optimal function is restored.

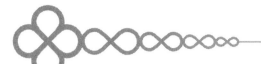

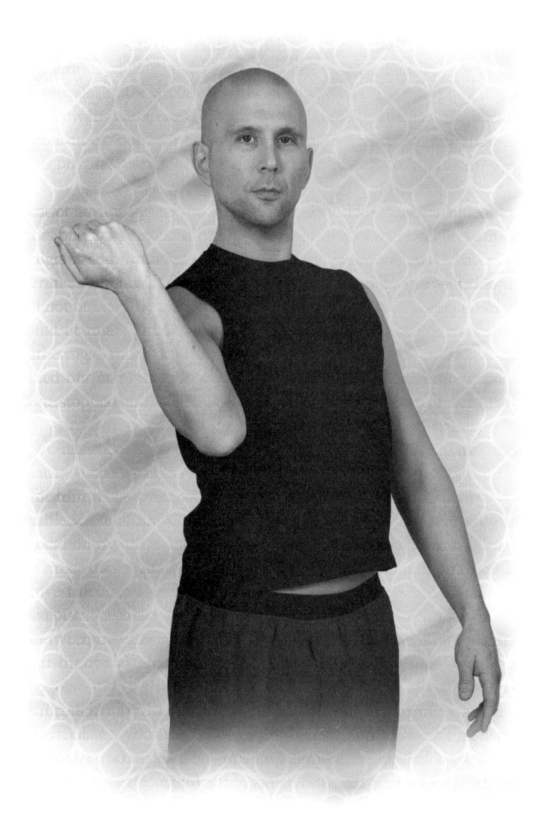

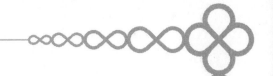

Crown Down and Heart Apart

The theory of becoming Free to Move is based on Intu-Flow (the joint mobility "wing" of the Circular Strength Training System). This motor development principle works from head to toe, core to periphery, bones to skin.

The first two principles relate to how we are genetically programmed due to the organized pattern of physical growth and motor control development called the cephalocaudal-proximodistal trend, which can be understood as moving from head to toe, core to periphery.

> Normal neurophysiologic growth and development of infants follow two principles. According to the cephalocaudal principle, development spreads over the body from head to foot. This means that improvement in structure and function comes first in the head region, then in the trunk, and last in the leg region.

According to the proximodistal principle, development proceeds from near to far — outward from the central axis of the body toward the extremities. In the fetus, the head and trunk are fairly well developed before the rudimentary limb buds appear. Gradually the arm buds lengthen and develop into hands and fingers. Functionally, babies can use their arms before their hands and can use their hands as a unit before they can control the movements of the fingers.

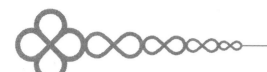

However, these principles do not "switch off" genetically after infancy. They remain "highways" for neurophysiologic growth and development in teenagers, adults, and seniors. (Vincent, E. L., and P. C. Martin. *Human Psychological Development.* Ronald, 1961.) These principles have guided motor skill acquisition curricula for prominent educational institutions such as the St. Petersburg Institute of Physical Culture (Russia), the Imperial Society for Teachers of Dancing (United Kingdom), and the Classic Homeopathic Research Center (India).

Matching skill acquisition training with the genetic process for improving the smoothness and accuracy of movements allows for rapid, precise skill acquisition.

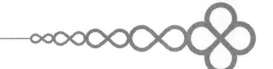

"Wash the Inner Bag"
XXIV

When myofascia is pulling too tightly or is too loose, the joint it acts upon can become dysfunctional as well. In order to begin training, we must completely reprogram movement involving that joint first locally and then integrate it globally.

In a state of dysfunctional motor coordination, one of the most common responses of the motor control center is to collapse the space between the joint. The smooth working of a joint requires the synergistic interaction of both the inner bag and the outer bag. If the outer bag is dysfunctional, it cannot properly support the inner bag, and it may collapse as a result. This closing of the joint spacing then becomes a part of the dysfunctional pattern that must be addressed first and foremost in any athletic program.

> If each joint is not decompressed and mobilized (in a specific sequence), the joints will not receive the nutrition and lubrication critical for healthy performance. They will not be able to ship out toxins. Joint salts can progress to calcifications. Adhesions can form, restricting range of motion and power. This degeneration of the connective tissue accelerates the aging process, resulting in dry, brittle joint surfaces, and significantly increases the risk of sudden, acute injury.

During every action involving resistance (including propulsion through gravity), a shock wave travels up from the point of contact throughout the body. When working efficiently, each joint individually and

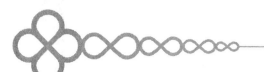

collectively behaves as a shock absorber. The shock wave will cause a slight, temporary compression but then automatically decompress like a spring. In contrast, a dysfunctional joint compresses as the shock wave hits it but cannot spring back to the proper spacing. This results in extra pressure on the tissues in the joint capsule. Such additional pressure leads to a host of common athletic injuries, such as epicondylitis; bursitis; knee, ankle, and hip strain; rotator cuff impingement; and spinal disc bulging and herniation, as well as an array of referred painful conditions such as neck stingers, radiculopathy, and sciatica.

>Adding athletic resistance over a compressed joint results in greater joint dysfunction and communicates further dysfunction to both proximal and distal joints adjacent to it as well as far from the local site.

Your mobility practice in Circular Strength Training decompresses the joint capsule of each joint as well as washes the inner bag with ground substance to return its natural resilience, elasticity, and shock-absorbent quality.

THE PROGRESSION OF PHYSICAL VIBRANCE

Your Circular Strength Training practice of mobility takes you through a specific process to:

- **Recover** basic ranges of motion (cardinal ranges and circles)
- **Coordinate** greater sophistication in mobility (infinities and diagonal infinities)
- **Refine** motor development in highly sophisticated movement (clovers and waves)

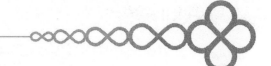

Below is a diagram for tracking the quadrants of movement up to clovers.

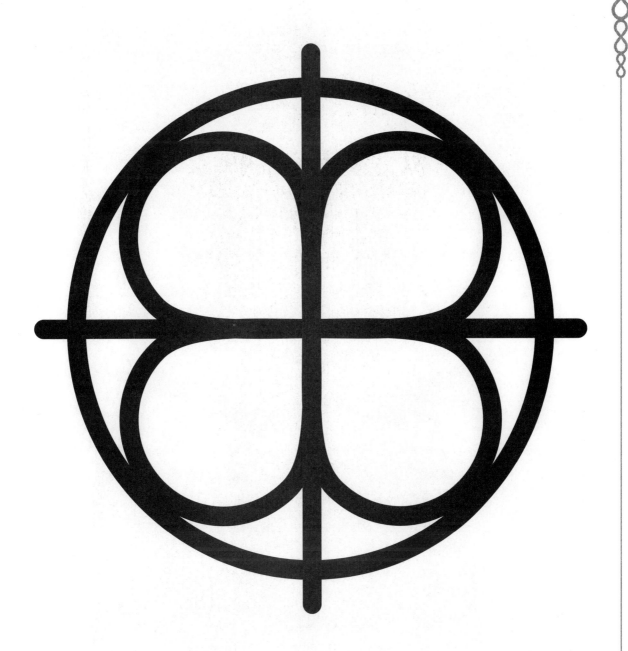

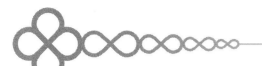

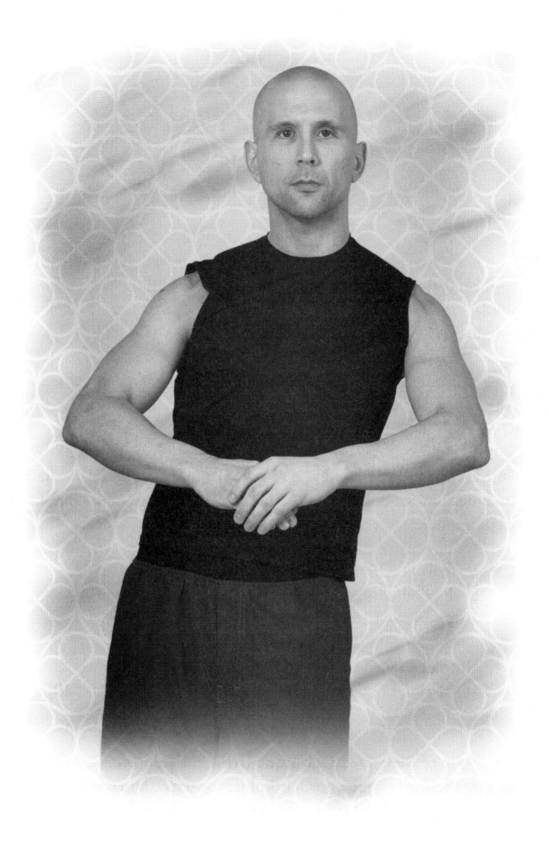

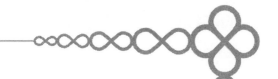

Intuitive Training

This ongoing process allows you to have 100% of the benefits from mobility because it's governed by your subjective experience of movement. This protocol I developed due to a need to protect my genetically challenged connective tissue from harm is called Intuitive Training.

Intuitive Training is very simple, but can feel challenging because of the many social, psychological, and energetic disconnects from your body. We can't move what we don't love.

Intuitive Training develops the ability to differentiate form, exertion, and discomfort subjectively, and then uses that knowledge as the determinant factor in progressive resistance:

- **Rate of perceived exertion (RPE):** The subjective evaluation of one's effort level based upon a scale of 1–10; 10 being the hardest one has ever worked

- **Rate of perceived discomfort (RPD):** The subjective evaluation of one's pain level based on a scale of 1–10; 10 being the worst pain one has ever experienced

- **Rate of perceived technique (RPT):** The subjective evaluation of one's mechanical performance based on a scale of 1–10; 10 being the best possible form

Technique is a bowl. Discomfort is a crack in the bowl. Effort is the water coming out of the faucet. If your technique is high enough (greater than or equal to 8) and your discomfort is low enough (less than or equal to 3), you can hold even an RPE of 10 for as long as your stamina, strength, and endurance allow.

First your stamina, strength, and endurance will diminish as the body protects itself from injury by the mechanism we call fatigue. As fatigue engages, technique diminishes. As technique diminishes, we no longer have the bowl to hold the fluid force of our effort, and discomfort increases. As discomfort increases, the potential for injury amplifies — since the degree of "poor" technique is actually a technique itself but unknown, unpredictable, unrepeatable, and potentially hazardous.

We always leak effort. In other words, when creating sufficient adaptation stress, we never have a technique of 10 and a discomfort of 0. There is always a degree of water rushing out of the faucet, splashing out of the bowl, slipping through the cracks. We play a game of maximizing what we can catch, minimizing what we lose. With an RPT >= 8 and an RPD <= 3, we can sufficiently hold an RPE of 6+.

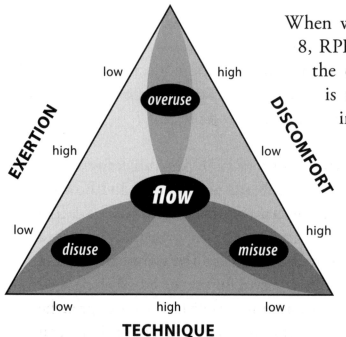

When we can sustain an RPT >= 8, RPD <= 3, and RPE >= 6 over the course of three sessions, it is time to increase a variable in the protocol: frequency, intensity, speed, density, volume, complexity, and so on.

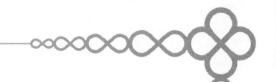

Understanding Pain

Contributed by Kathryn Woodall, D.C.

"Pain is important; how we evade it, how we succumb to it, how we deal with it, how we transcend it."
Audre Lorde

Pain is a form of communication between our body and our awareness. Too often we fail to see it as such and instead of listening to what it is saying, we do all that we can to ignore it or to get it to shut up. Can you imagine what would happen if any other loved ones were talking to us and we chose to ignore them or asked them to shut up? If ignored regularly perhaps they would nag at us. Or thinking that we hadn't heard, perhaps they would become more of a pain about trying to get our attention. If we told them to shut up they might recruit others to talk to us in order to prove their point. (The shoulder pain went away, but now the elbow hurts.) However, even when we do listen, sometimes we misunderstand what is being said.

A question that is often presented to me is, "How do I know when to give an injury or pain time to see if it heals by itself, and how do I know when I need to see my health care team about it?" I'd like to offer some basic information about pain that you may use as a guideline. The information provided is not so that you can make a self-diagnosis because that can be a very dangerous and slippery road to travel upon. But having at least a faint idea of how to interpret the possible things being said when your body sends you a pain signal can

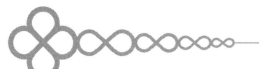

be useful. If you hear it when it is whispering instead of ignore it until it is screaming, you might be able to avoid the injury or illness that can come from delayed attention.

There are two main types of pain: acute and chronic. Acute pain is predictable and within the range of what is considered appropriate for the injury or illness that is present. While it describes the sharp and sudden pain due to a broken arm, acute pain can also be used to describe the tooth that is aching now but that was fine only a couple of days ago. Chronic pain falls outside of the range of what is typically predictable and common for an injury or illness. An example would be a sprained ankle that still hurts three months later or a headache that has been occurring once a month for the last six months.

The two types of pain can be approached differently. Let's look at acute pain first.

Acute pain that occurs without a known cause is something that you should *always* visit your doctor about. Infections, cancers, blood clots, heart attacks, bleeding ulcers, and other serious conditions may be the source of unknown acute pain, and waiting around to see if "maybe it will just go away" is a bad idea for this type of pain.

Acute pain that you know the source of is more common, and while sometimes it will require the help of your doctor, at other times it may not. There are obvious things that should land you in the emergency room as soon as possible, such as a bone sticking through skin, skin deformity (the bone isn't sticking through the skin but is causing a bulge or a cavity where normally one does not exist), inability to move an arm or a leg, loss of consciousness, or a cut that won't stop bleeding. For things not as obvious, the following two lists can serve as a guide. They are by no means all inclusive and if there is ever any doubt whether medical attention is needed, it is always best to seek it.

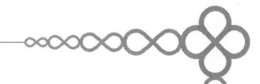

May be a minor injury that will heal on its own:

- A cut that stops bleeding and is superficial [The delayed development of pus or heat at the site of the cut may indicate an infection, and medical attention should then be sought.]
- Light swelling at a point of impact
- A "tweaked joint" with the only symptom present being pain that settles at or below a 6 or a 7 (on a scale of 1–10, with 10 being the most pain you have ever felt and 1 being mild discomfort) quickly after the initial tweak [If the pain stays at a 6 or a 7 for more than 24 hours, it then becomes an injury that may need medical attention.]
- A surface abrasion such as a skinned knee or elbow
- Mild bruising at the location of pain with either very minor or no swelling
- A "turned/sprained ankle" only when there is mild to no swelling, no pops or clicks were felt or heard, no bruising is present, and the ankle is not more or less movable than prior to the "turn"
- A charley horse or other spasm that subsides with massage, rest, or stretching [If this is a one-time event it can be considered minor. However, if it is repeated over the course of days or weeks, seeking a cause with the help of your health care team is advised.]

Definitely needs medical attention:

- A pop or snap followed by pain, swelling, or both [Depending upon the area of the body, this might indicate a torn meniscus, torn ligament, torn tendon, herniated disc, or broken bone.]
- On a scale of 1–10 (10 being the most pain you have ever felt and 1 being mild discomfort), pain staying at or above an 8 for more than a few seconds to minutes

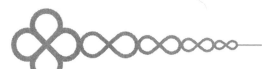

- On the above 1–10 scale, pain at a level of 6–7 for longer than 24 hours
- Pain that increases instead of decreases after 24 hours
- Pain accompanied by heat at or beside the area
- Bruising occurring after very light or no impact
- Excessive swelling (so much that joint motion is altered)
- A grinding sound is produced on use of the injured area [If grinding occurs, stop moving the area immediately because a broken bone may be present.]
- Pain accompanied by vomiting, diarrhea, profuse sweating, or loss of bowel/bladder function [This could indicate damage to an internal organ, internal bleeding, or pressure upon the spinal cord.]
- A cut that is deep enough to show fatty tissue, muscle, tendon, nerve, or bone
- An inability to move an otherwise movable body part
- An otherwise immovable body part displaying motion
- Pain that radiates down an arm or leg, around the rib cage, or up or down the spine
- Swelling that "pits" (when you push your finger into it, the indentation remains for longer than a few seconds) [This can indicate cardiovascular problems.]
- Numbness [Think of numbness as your body giving you the silent treatment. Just like in any other conversation, at the point that the other party is so fed up that it won't talk to you, things are in a serious state.]
- Any of the "minor injury" list that persists for longer than expected or has increased symptoms [Swelling should be mostly gone within 1–3 days, cuts should heal in 1–2 weeks, a lightly sprained ankle should be fully functional and discomfort free in about 2 weeks, bruises should be gone in about 2 weeks.]

Then there is the acute pain where you aren't positive about the cause but feel like it *might* have been something you did. An example would be waking up with neck discomfort and wondering if you "just slept wrong." The rule of thumb in order for this type of pain to be considered minor is that it should go away within 3 days at the most, the pain or discomfort should not increase, the pain goes away when you stop doing the activity you believe caused it (and that activity isn't something that you have always done but suddenly suspect as a culprit), other symptoms should not appear, and it should not continue to come and go over the course of the following weeks or months. If any of that rule of thumb is not true, then it is time to consult your health care team because the pain you are experiencing falls into the "unknown cause" category and needs to be investigated immediately.

Chronic pain is a slightly different story, and determining when to see your doctor and when not to is a bit more difficult. If you don't know the cause of the chronic pain, then it is definitely time to see your health care team to find out the cause. If you have a diagnosis and understand your condition, then you should ask your doctor what signs and symptoms warrant another visit. If you have been diagnosed with a condition that is associated with chronic pain, it might also be useful to obtain a second, third, or even fourth opinion to confirm the diagnosis. Doctors are human, and there is so much to know and learn about the human body that no one person will ever fully grasp all of it. Just because the person (or possibly specialty) you are currently seeing doesn't have an answer for you it doesn't mean that someone else (or another specialty) won't. Things are being discovered and new treatments are being tried all the time. Ask your health care team what you can do to minimize the progression of your condition, what you can do to improve your health as much as possible, if there are things you definitely should not do, and if there are things you definitely should do, and take this book to them to see if it is safe for you to implement the techniques discussed.

While pain often occurs at the sight of injury or illness, it can also radiate along the course of a nerve. If there is a herniated disc in the neck, a person may experience a dull ache in the neck while she feels like her entire arm is on fire. The arm itself is basically fine except that the nerve that serves it is highly inflamed. An overly tight muscle, a bony protrusion, or a tumor placing pressure on the soft tissue around a nerve can cause the same type of problem as a herniated disc. If you are experiencing radiating pain you should see your health care provider so that you can get started with a therapy program that is appropriate for your diagnosis.

Referred pain is pain that is unexpectedly experienced at a site away from its source. One form of this occurs when one joint is not functioning well (from injury or fatigue) but it is the neighboring joint that experiences the pain. An example would be if a person started having knee pain but an examination and X-ray didn't find anything wrong with the knee. The doctor might then continue with her exam and find that a previously sprained ankle wasn't fully rehabilitated, and although it isn't hurting, the ankle's altered motion is causing the pain at the knee. Trigger points (hyperirritable spots in taut bands of muscle) in one muscle have also been shown to cause pain in a different muscle.

Another form of referred pain occurs when an injured or diseased organ causes pain in a muscle at a distance from the organ. The most well-known example is a heart attack referring pain to the chest and left arm. While there are a few theories as to why this sometimes occurs, the most common is that the organ and the muscular area it refers pain to are linked neurologically. This is called viscerosomatic convergence.

Regardless of cause, people experiencing referred pain almost always think it is a problem with the muscle or joint where they feel the pain and don't realize that another organ is at play. Because the quality of pain can range from a dull ache to a sharp, stabbing pain, the quality

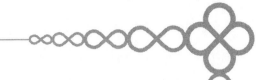

of pain alone will not hint at the source. The muscles in the area where pain is showing up can be tight and tender, and can even restrict joint motion and function. Sometimes there will be tenderness if the area where the other organ sits is touched, and sometimes there will not.

So how do you know if it is referred pain from some other organ or if there is a problem with the muscles in the area where you are feeling pain? Usually you don't without an examination from a qualified health care practitioner. However, there is a slight problem with that too. There are lots of people who go to see their doctor and are diagnosed with a musculoskeletal problem but told to come back if the problem continues. The problem does continue but patients don't go back because what the doctor recommended didn't help them after the first visit. Therefore the doctor couldn't do further testing to rule out other problems and find the actual cause. I'm adding the following list of common referral patterns not as a way for you to diagnose yourself but so that you can be aware that the patterns exist and that they need to be considered if you are not responding to treatment as expected. The following is not an all-inclusive list but does cover the most common patterns seen:

Adrenal glands
- Lower rib cage

Aorta (the large artery that leaves the heart and runs down through the abdomen)
- Between the shoulder blades
- Chest
- Neck
- Midline abdominal region
- Lower back
- The most common reason for referred pain from the aorta is an aneurysm (a ballooned-out section of the artery, which can burst) or a dissection after trauma (the artery is torn and blood is leaking out).

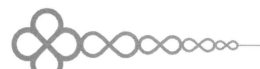

Appendix
- Typically refers to the umbilical area (belly button)
- Occasionally refers to the right shoulder
- Lower back
- Pelvis

Diaphragm (This is a muscle that is being included because it can be inflamed by a number of organs.)
- Either or both shoulders
- Neck

Ears
- Jaw

Esophagus
- Chest
- Throat
- Neck (especially with acid reflux)

Eyes (including visual problems)
- Back of the head (may cause headaches affecting more than just the back of the head)
- Upper neck

Gallbladder
- Right shoulder
- Right scapular region (shoulder blade area)
- Midline abdominal region

Heart
- Left shoulder
- Chest (While it is common for men to experience chest pain before and during a heart attack, women may not have any chest pain before or during a heart attack [1])
- Less commonly the right shoulder

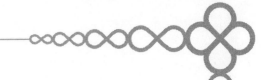

- Between the shoulder blades (more common in females than the chest or shoulder)
- Neck (more common in females than in males)

Kidneys
- Lower rib cage
- Pain into the lower back and pelvis if one or more ureters are involved (such as with passing a kidney stone)
- May refer pain to the midline abdominal region
- Hips via inflammation of the psoas muscle and its innervation (and possibly achy knees via hip function)

Large intestine
- Often it refers pain to the midline abdominal region
- Lower back
- Lower rib cage
- Pelvis

Liver
- Right shoulder
- Right side of the mid back
- The neck via inflammation of the diaphragm — usually the right side of the neck
- Midline abdominal region

Lungs
- Either shoulder
- Neck
- Between the shoulder blades

Pancreas
- Lower aspect of the mid back
- The left shoulder via inflammation of the diaphragm
- The neck via inflammation of the diaphragm — usually the left side of the neck

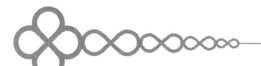

- Midline abdominal region

Reproductive organs (ovaries, testes, uterus, prostrate)
- Lower back
- Pelvis
- Thighs

Small intestine
- Typically pain would be felt midline in the abdominal region
- Occasionally there is referral to the chest (An ulcer will sometimes refer pain to the chest.)
- Pain may be referred to the lower back

Spleen
- Left shoulder
- Left scapular area (shoulder blade)
- Left mid back
- Midline abdominal region

Stomach
- Mid back
- Chest
- The left shoulder via inflammation of the diaphragm
- Midline abdominal region

Teeth
- Jaw
- Neck
- Face

Thyroid gland
- Neck
- Throat

- Can inflame the surrounding tissues enough to cause radiating pain down either arm

Urinary bladder
- Pelvis

Pain is not a bad thing, and it is not your body betraying you. It is a warning system and a form of communication attempting to tell you that something is not right and needs attention. With the exception of direct trauma, pain is often the last thing to show up in an injury or disease process and the first thing to go once treatment has begun. Your body is extremely adept at compensating for a problem, and typically it will have tried every compensation it can before it tries to get your attention via discomfort or pain. Love your pain. It is a gift trying to teach you something about yourself that you were unaware of until it spoke up.

[1] Vaccarino, V., Parson, L., Every, N.R., Barron, H., et al. *Sex-Based Differences in Early Mortality After Myocardial Infarction*, New England Journal of Medicine 341, no. 4 (1999): 217-25

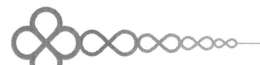

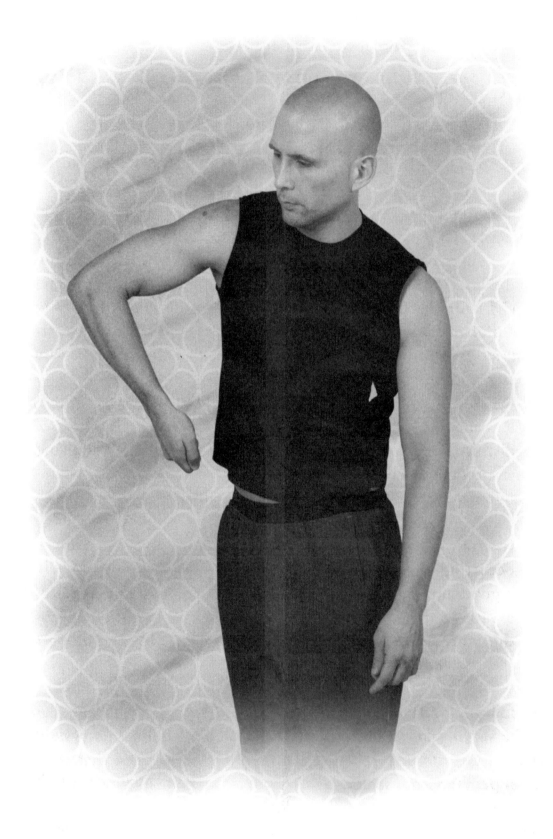

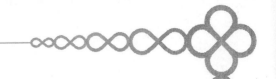

Understanding Snap, Crackle, Pop!

Contributed by Jarlo Ilano, L.P.T.

Many types of sounds are generated from our bodies in the various motions we perform, whether as part of specific exercise or simply when getting up in the morning. Depending upon who you talk to, these sounds are either to be avoided like the plague, glossed over, or sought after like the Holy Grail.

The distinct nature of the sounds, in general, also gives some insight into their physiological underpinnings. What exactly is happening when you hear a click, pop, snap, clunk, or grind?

In truth, it can be quite difficult to say with great accuracy what is occurring, though we can make quality inferences — especially with a good amount of experience in the examination and assessment of a variety of individuals. Needless to say, the accuracy significantly diminishes if the health care provider is not present to both hear and feel the sounds as they are happening.

The following essay is a general exposition regarding the phenomenon of the varying noises drawn forth from the musculoskeletal system. These noises are distinct from the more obvious sounds that often accompany trauma, such as the tearing of a ligament or tendon, as in the expression "I blew my knee out," or the very loud sound of an Achilles tendon rupturing, or the cracking sound of a broken bone.

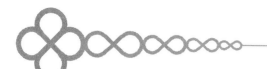

These are accompanied by significant pain and should of course be followed by immediate medical attention. Rather, this essay is meant to give insight into what is really happening as we hear the everyday sounds of these snaps, crackles, and pops!

The pop you sometimes hear when you move your body and stretch your back or "crack" your knuckles is from the fluid in your joints transforming into gas. This *synovial fluid* is located within the soft tissue that surrounds the movable joints in our body. The tissue is called a *joint capsule;* it is a closed system filled with fluid, so any deformation causes a change in pressure. As the joint capsule distends and increases in volume, the pressure decreases and bubbles form in the liquid to eventually burst and turn into gas. This is called *cavitation.* "A radiographic negative shadow appears within the joint with the density of nitrogen ... The cavitation phenomenon suggests that the synovial fluid changes from a liquid to a gaseous state." (Greenman, 1996.)

This is why you cannot crack your knuckles again immediately after you have just cracked them. It's been found that it takes approximately 20 minutes for the pressure to normalize and the gas to absorb back into the fluid. For those sounds that emanate repeatedly with a certain motion, it would appear that they are not a result of this mechanism.

As for other sounds? This is where we can go awry. Debate from many perspectives can be very difficult to wade through; however, here are some of my interpretations. Repetitive clicks could be connective tissue out of its proper alignment or cartilaginous tissue damage such as torn meniscal flaps or other impairment. *Crepitus,* or crunching, is most likely tissue damage on the surface of your joints. This *chondral* tissue damage is what doctors are referring to when they advise arthritic patients that their knees are "bone on bone." The normally protective tissue is often worn down with age and misuse of the joints. Another sound, more like a "rip," can often be heard or felt as well. This is commonly scar tissue, which builds up like a callous after irritation

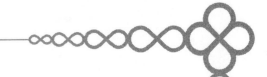

or damage. Depending on the situation, it can be beneficial or problematic.

The "clunk" is an interesting phenomenon. Often accompanying a feeling of a "shift" in the joints, it may or may not accompany the louder pop. This occurrence is generally acknowledged as a distinct entity. It may be a true *subluxation,* in which the joint is off axis (normal position) and a particular movement shifts it back on axis. This is a relatively controversial topic, but I think there is merit for this, particularly in the wrists, ankle, sacrum, and low lumbar spine. These sounds occur in what I would classify as *hypermobile* joints and the ones most in need of stabilization through neurological retraining of the surrounding musculature. The joint has also been termed *compressed* in that as it is off its anatomical axis, its motion is abnormally curtailed; thus the feeling that it is not moving freely. This compressed joint can also be from high muscular tone around the structure.

When a joint is stretched or manipulated, the joint capsule is distended and the stretch on the capsule stimulates *Type III joint mechanoreceptors,* which cause a neuroreflexive inhibition of surrounding muscles. In other words, the muscles around a joint that has been popped decrease in tone and become less tight. This appears to be the most suitable explanation for the relaxation and ease that we feel. Another theory is that various chemicals are released after a joint is stretched. These have been called *endogenous opiates;* thus the good feeling many people experience after a high-velocity thrust manipulation as employed by chiropractors, physical therapists, and other health care providers. As you can imagine, this can be quite addictive!

A relevant debate is whether these manipulations should be repeated, or even performed at all. Many people are advised that repeated cracking of the joints can lead to arthritis and other joint damage. Yet there are no definitive studies that prove damage from repeated popping of your joints. In fact, a study by Castellanos and Axelrod (1990) found that in their study group of 300 people, 74 who were described as "habitual knuckle

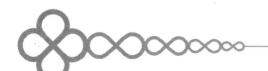
crackers" had no significant differences in the amount of joint damage. However, the researchers did find increased hand swelling and decreased grip strength, and advised against consistent knuckle cracking.

Can this study be applied to all joints in our body? Perhaps repetitive stimulation of the joint mechanoreceptors, discussed above, can lead to improper joint movement patterns, as the surrounding musculature is continually inhibited. Essentially, you become too relaxed. Also, it has been shown the chronic inflammation decreases tissue stability. And it is well known that repetitive overstretching can bring about inflammation.

Does this mean that we can do too much mobility training? Can the range of motion training we do have effects similar to those from overstretching or continually cracking our joints? What about those pops and clunks that happen not just when we quickly twist our backs but also when we exercise smoothly and slowly?

It is my opinion that the passive popping and cracking that occur in a normal range of motion (not a fast, jerky twitch or a twisting of our joints) are because of the higher muscular and fascial tension that often turns up in our tired and stressed bodies. Some days we move our arms in a circle and there is no sound, and other days after a hard day at work we stretch out and hear a pop. The tension is higher than normal and can pull upon the joint capsule more than usual and result in the noise. I believe this is sort of a natural "reset" that occurs to discharge some of the built-up tension. If you are moving smoothly and deliberately in your exercise and noise occurs, it is generally nothing to worry about.

Another common phenomenon is for a noise to change over time. It can become louder, more frequent, or less frequent; be accompanied by pain; or suddenly become pain-free. This is because the angles of pull and axes of motion can change with increased or decreased muscle strength and flexibility, and with other changes in soft tissue. It is not uncommon to observe the noises appearing and disappearing during the course of an exercise regimen as your body adapts and changes.

As to the issue of too much mobility training, I used to think that you could not do too much as long as you were engaging in pain-free smooth and steady exercise. However, Scott Sonnon wrote of the *training effect* that happens when practice moves beyond a certain threshold. It is no longer a joint mobility recovery and maintenance exercise but instead turns into a *conditioning* exercise that can reinforce the wrong adaptations. This isn't necessarily felt right away, but is often felt as delayed soreness the following morning or with decreased performance in the next exercise session. We should be aware of the fine line between practice and training. Five to 10 repetitions of exercises daily in a program such as Intu-Flow are most likely just fine; however, twice-daily sessions of a yoga and mobility program such as Ageless Mobility may be right on the edge of too much. As always, it is relative to individuals and their current status in their physical regimen.

I would suggest that you monitor your daily condition and exercises using the CST Intuitive Protocol and assess your ratings of discomfort as you continue your daily practice. And if you hear pops or a clunk, as long as you are not in pain, simply continue your active range-of-motion exercises.

Dynamic range of motion such as presented in Intu-Flow and other therapeutic exercise will serve to prevent joint compression and enhance muscular strength (both neurological and structural) and flexibility. So with intelligent and consistent daily practice, rather than experience the sounds as a goal, hindrance, or bane, you will understand they are just a normal part of regaining your freedom of movement.

Greenman, Philip. *Principles of Manual Medicine*, 2nd ed., Lippincott Williams & Wilkins, 1996, p.100.

Castellanos J., and D. Axelrod. "Effect of Habitual Knuckle Cracking on Hand Function," *Annals of the Rheumatic Diseases*, 49(5):308–9, 1990.

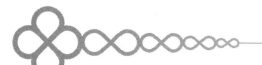

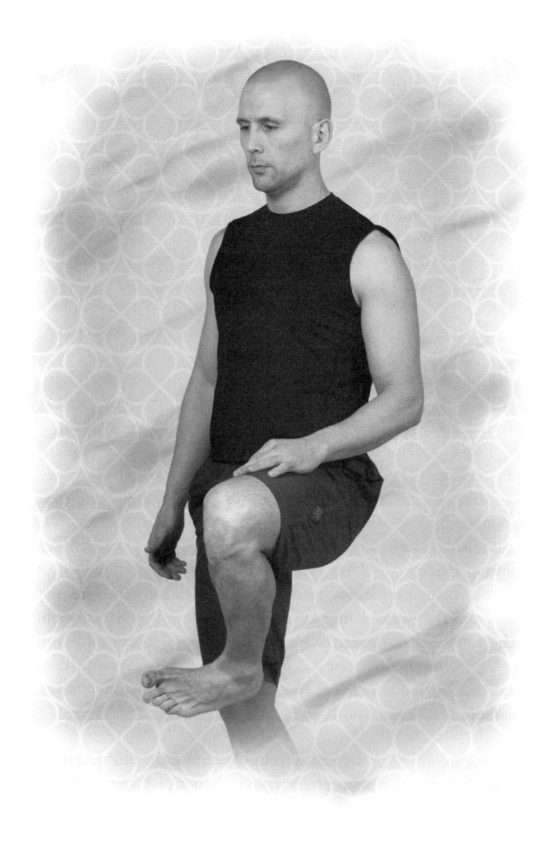

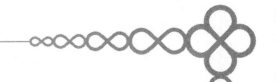

Prehab, Rehab, Posthab

Contributed by Jarlo Ilano, L.P.T.

*P**rehab**, or "prehabilitation," is a term first coined 20 years ago by Tom House, a well-known pitching coach who was disturbed by how many of his athletes were sidelined by rotator cuff problems. He felt that many of these injuries could be prevented, and suggested exercises to strengthen his pitchers' weak areas. The term soon spread and has been applied in many other sports and training regimens, with the common goal of injury prevention.*

Circular Strength Training's particular brand of prehab is intertwined throughout the system. The flagship Intu-Flow program was designed to systematically engage every active joint in your body to promote full musculoskeletal health. Full freedom of movement is a key step to proper prehabilitation. Yet rather than ending there, the concept of prehab is consistent in the training regimen even as the intensity increases and the work changes toward more specific goals. Inherent in each biomechanical exercise are components for joint health and prevention of injury. Because CST is a "health first" system, each segment of a particular training protocol includes compensations and awareness of total body health.

Rehabilitation is the prescribed course of care in the health care process as directed by your physician and physical therapist. Dependent upon a patient's particular condition and his or her individual response, rehab programs draw upon the significant knowledge base and experience

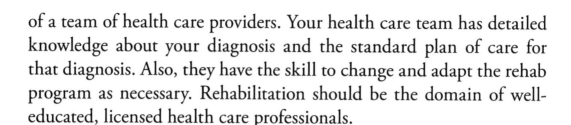

of a team of health care providers. Your health care team has detailed knowledge about your diagnosis and the standard plan of care for that diagnosis. Also, they have the skill to change and adapt the rehab program as necessary. Rehabilitation should be the domain of well-educated, licensed health care professionals.

Posthab refers to the physical training you undergo after you are cleared from the rehabilitation process by your health care providers. After you meet distinct goals and following a proper assessment of your current status, your physician or therapist often prescribes a home exercise program, or directs you to a particular physical training regimen. It is not uncommon for physicians to recommend yoga or strength training to their patients, either as a transition to the patient's choice of recreational activity or simply as a healthy physical practice that encourages full recovery. It is at this point that many people engage the services of a fitness professional to help them toward further goals. Clients should feel comfortable that their trainer is aware of their posthab status and can appropriately individualize their program.

The distinction between prehab, rehab, and posthab may be difficult to see since many of the exercises and activities appear to be similar. The exercises may be quite alike, but often the intent, sequencing, and intensity of the movement activities are specific to the patient's status and condition. The primary distinction is whether or not your health care provider is involved. When he is, he is responsible for your total condition and, as such, is (along with yourself) the primary decision maker for your course of exercise, especially if you are recovering from a surgical intervention. A personal trainer has no business recommending any program that differs from your surgeon's postoperative instructions.

An enlightening example contrasts the use of the foam rollers by personal trainers and by health care providers. Foam rollers are cylindrical, dense foam devices that are used in many gyms and fitness centers. The various exercises and methods of use were taken from techniques originally employed by health care providers. In recent years they seem to have trickled down to personal trainers, who are employing them with clients. This is not automatically a bad thing, as many people would swear to have experienced great benefit.

> However, the concern is that personal trainers are not adequately trained in the full scope of these techniques, especially as they are to be integrated in a rehabilitation regimen. Very often the trainers pick a few exercises of the overall method and apply them to every client. Their training is of course not as extensive as a health care provider's. If it were, then they would be licensed rehabilitation professionals as well!

I have used foam rollers extensively for many years in my physical therapy practice. They are a great tool. They can be used for soft tissue release (as many personal trainers seem to use them for), but also for joint manipulation, proprioceptive training, and specific breathing exercise. Foam rollers, Swiss balls, and balance discs were originally employed by pediatric physical therapists in the treatment of children with delayed developmental disorders. And there are many contraindications, both absolute and conditional, that need to be known before they are used in a person's rehabilitation program. With this in mind, does it seem likely that a personal trainer is as qualified as a health care provider to use this tool?

> It may seem harmless, as we see their use in the gym, but it can be an example of the line being crossed by some personal trainers. Many attempt to dip into the tools of rehab for new and exotic ways to impress their clients. Rather than tread into this possibly risky water, trainers should do their best within their particular scope of knowledge. There are more than enough variations of exercise in the fitness field to keep clients and trainers busy for a long time.

Circular Strength Training instructors are trained in the CST system not to be rehabilitation professionals, but to be fitness professionals.

They are well versed in providing programs for clients to improve their freedom of movement. Whereas a health care provider may properly indicate a diagnosis of bicipital tendonitis (inflammation of the biceps tendon), CST instructors should not presume to do the same. Instead, these instructors should work within the framework of their training in a way that is consistent with CST principles, and within the context that clients have been cleared by their health care providers. For example, an instructor may choose to have the client work on a variety of upper-back and shoulder circles along with different biomechanical exercises to strengthen particular areas.

The distinctions between prehab, rehab, and posthab are important not just for the sake of proper terminology, but because of the necessity to place our health first. Every activity we engage in either promotes or hinders our health, and we should place a high premium on our personal health and well being. This, of course, includes a sound daily physical fitness regimen. Along with that, it also requires us to be thoughtful and intelligent about the process. We need to be aware of when it is necessary to consult health care professionals and engage in the plan of care that they prescribe. The differences separating prehab, rehab, and posthab are part of the careful and smart attitude we should all have when taking care of ourselves.

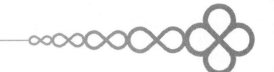

Aging: The Process of Losing Complexity

As we age, we strive to make life simpler and simpler in an attempt to reduce it to its most essential characteristics. Unfortunately, doing so accelerates the aging process. Professor Mario Kyriazis, medical adviser to the British Longevity Society, explains: "If you want to live a long and healthy life, quite the worst thing you can do is to avoid stress to either mind or body. Aging is due to the loss of complexity in our system, and the way to boost complexity is to challenge the system. If you want to live long and healthily, don't settle into routines." (Bonsor, Sacha. "Bad stress, good stress: Coping with pressure can be a challenge with both physical and psychological benefits." The Times Online. September 20, 2005)

Aging — this gradual loss of complexity — results from the deterioration of an organism caused by strain (an over-abundance or under-abundance of stress), and eventually ends with loss of the animating force: an event we call death. (Mark P. Mattson, Wenzhen Duan, Ruqian Wan, Zhihong Guo. *"Activation of Neuroprotective Stress Response Pathways by Dietary and Behavioral Manipulations."* NeuroRx. 2004 January; 1(1): 111–116.)

Albert Einstein wrote, *"Life should be simple, and no simpler."* And yet, we are inundated with products and systems which proclaim themselves to be "the ultimate in simplicity". That hyperbole plays into our impulse to make things easier to understand, catering only to what we already know and do. This doesn't aid your fitness, and by definition it accelerates the aging process.

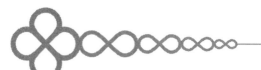

Think of it this way:

- The simpler the movement, the less movement you must do.

- The more you repeat the simple movement, the more conditioned that simple movement becomes.

- The more conditioned that simple movement becomes, the more you repeat it.

- The more that simple movements are repeated, the less that complex movements are attempted.

- The less complex movements attempted, the less stimulation of growth.

- The less stimulation of growth, the faster you age.

THE NERVOUS SYSTEM CRAVES COMPLEXITY!

We all feel the compulsion to prefer simplicity in our routines. We prefer mindlessness because the complexity of our lives is compounded by stress, children, work, projects, and the endless sea of daily surprises that life throws our way. Who wouldn't want to make the sanctuary of exercise as simple as possible?

We should. But we should take care to make it as Einstein suggested: **simple, but no simpler.** As you can see with the Intu-Flow Longevity System, exercise can be incredibly simple. However, an intelligent design allows you to improve your complexity as you master it.

We need to keep challenging our nervous system. We need to keep improving our complexity. We need to attempt new skills where we are not expert, where we are again only beginners. We must return

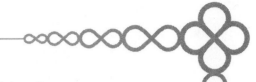

again and again to that stumbling, bumbling chuckle of incompetence which is the hallmark of the rapid learning curve of children.

This isn't to say that children learn better than adults. That notion goes against everything logical about complex systems. It's just that, when we hit a critical threshold we have a tendency to try to make life as simple as possible, and we often drift too far into over-simplification.

Bruce Lee wrote that before formal training a punch is just a punch. When training begins, and for the first few years, a punch is much more than a punch. After substantial experience, a punch becomes just a punch again.

It's a great thing to master a subject, but once mastered it's time to move on to another subject, or to a deeper, more complex aspect of the same subject. To avoid accelerating the aging process, we must forever thrust ourselves again and again into beginner's mode, and we must discover how much more there is to a subject before it becomes simple again.

The Intu-Flow Longevity System, presented in this book, offers a simple template which allows you to improve in complexity with practice.

COMBINED MOVEMENTS: LESSONS FROM PHYSIOTHERAPY

Part of my Russian experience involved learning a method of active self-physiotherapy where the body was taken through different ranges of motion to determine dysfunction — or "hitches" in movement — where limitations were found.

We don't feel this loss of complexity in basic ranges of movement, because we use them every day. However, when we increase the sophistication of movement by combining different actions together (such as flexion with rotation, or the multiple actions of one joint with

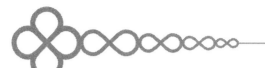

that of another joint) we can experience hidden restrictions in our movement and crepitus (snaps, cracks and pops) in our joints.

By increasing our movement sophistication we send lubrication and nutrition to the joint, and we have the potential to "scour" the joint and restore free mobility.

Motor sophistication in the Intu-Flow Longevity System happens through the following process:

1. **Ranges:** i.e. moving from front to rear, or from right to left.

2. **Circles:** i.e. continuing from front to right, to rear, to left, and back to the front once again.

3. **(Cardinal) Infinities:** dividing the basic circles in half (front and rear; right and left), we now have "figure eight" movements; i.e. moving left, front, right, left, rear, right, left.

4. **Diagonal Infinities:** dividing the basic circle into four quadrants (front left, front right, rear right, rear left), we now have "figure eight" movements diagonally across the quadrants; i.e. moving left, front, rear, right, left.

5. **Clovers:** we can now move through each quadrant in sequence; i.e. front, left, right, front, rear, right, left, rear, front.

6. **Waves:** movement between multiple joints fluidly; i.e. shoulder lifts, then elbow, then wrists, then fingers, like a rolling wave of the ocean.

If you follow these diagrams, you will gain a basic understanding of how we cultivate this innate grace through Intu-Flow.

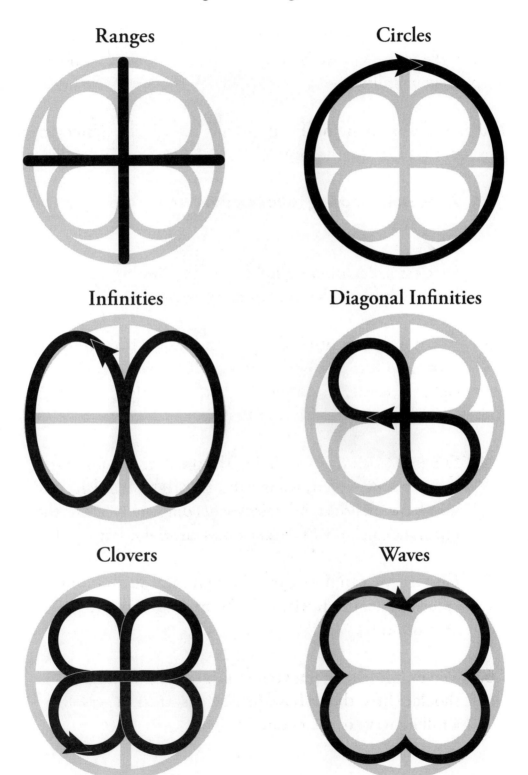

Ranges

Circles

Infinities

Diagonal Infinities

Clovers

Waves

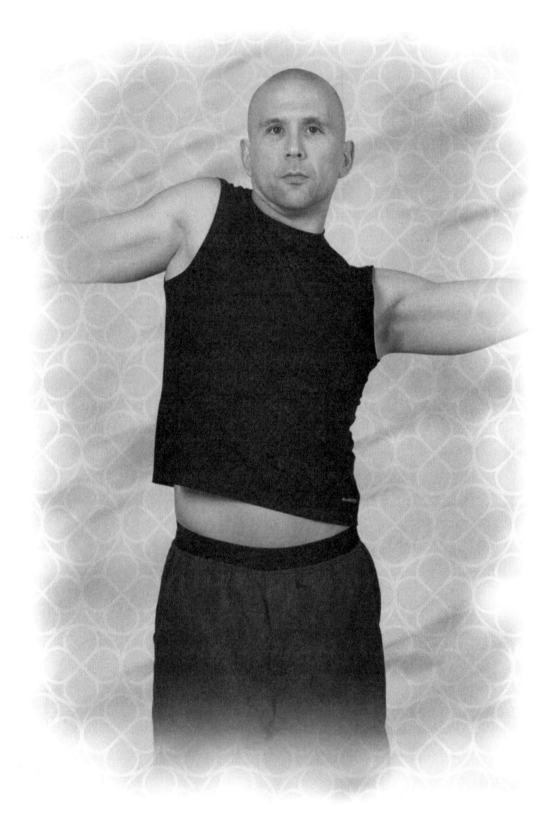

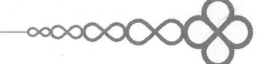

Exercises

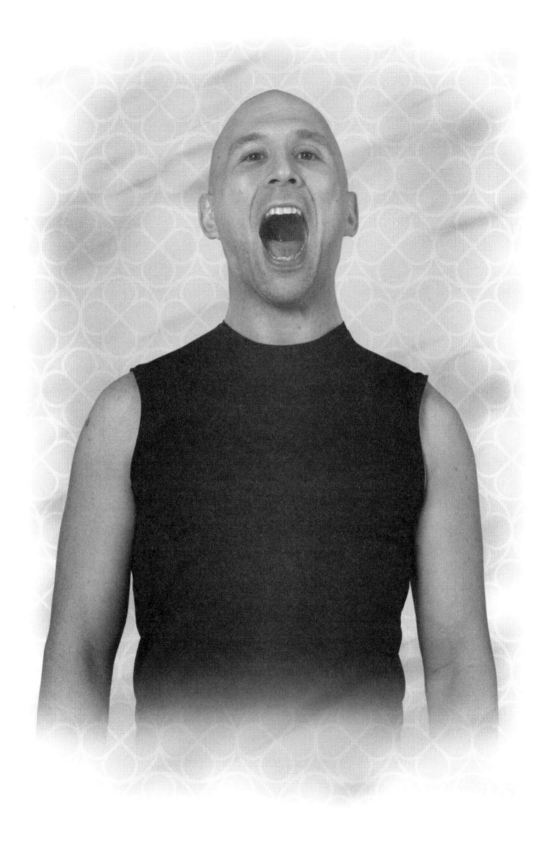

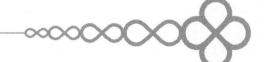

Jaw
Head
Face

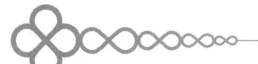

When not Free to Move from lack of prehabilitative movement due to stress, trauma, fear, overuse, underuse, or misuse, the following issues may result:

- Temporomandibular disorders
- Prognathism
- Face pain
- Bruxism
- Dislocated jaw
- Osteoarthritis

Common mental and emotional issues faced as a result of the area not being Free to Move:

- Anger
- Resentment — wanting to speak up but holding your tongue
- Desire for revenge
- Feeling you are biting off more than you can chew

Common organ referral affecting sensory-motor function of the area:

- The ear can refer pain to and affect the function of the jaw.
- The eyes (including visual problems) can refer pain to the back of the head and cause neck tightness.
- Dental problems can refer pain to the jaw, face, and neck.
- Dental problems can also alter function of the jaw and neck.

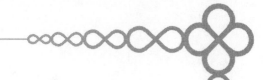

Several exercises will help you become Free to Move again:

1. **Ranges**
   a. Open
   b. Closed
   c. Right
   d. Left

2. **Circles**
   a. Open – right – closed – left
   b. Open – left – closed – right

3. **Infinities**
   a. Left – open – right – left – closed – right
   b. Right – open – left – right – closed – left
   c. Open – right – closed – open – left – closed
   d. Closed – right – open – closed – left – open

4. **Diagonal infinities**
   a. Open – right – left – closed – open
   b. Closed – left – right – open – closed
   c. Open – left – right – closed – open
   d. Closed – right – left – open – closed

5. **Clovers**
   a. Open – right – left – open – closed – left – right – closed
   b. Closed – right – left – closed – open – left – right – open

RANGES

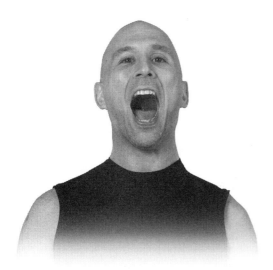

Open

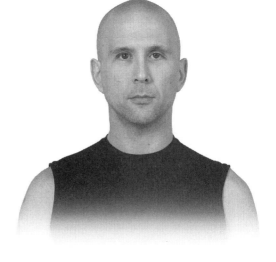

Closed

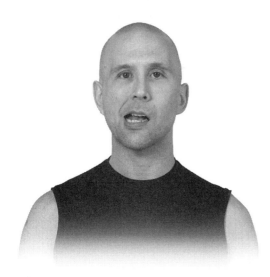

Right

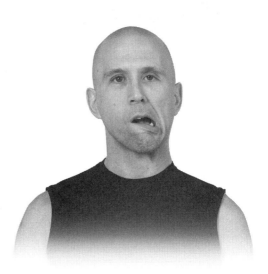

Left

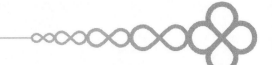

CIRCLES
Open – right – closed – left

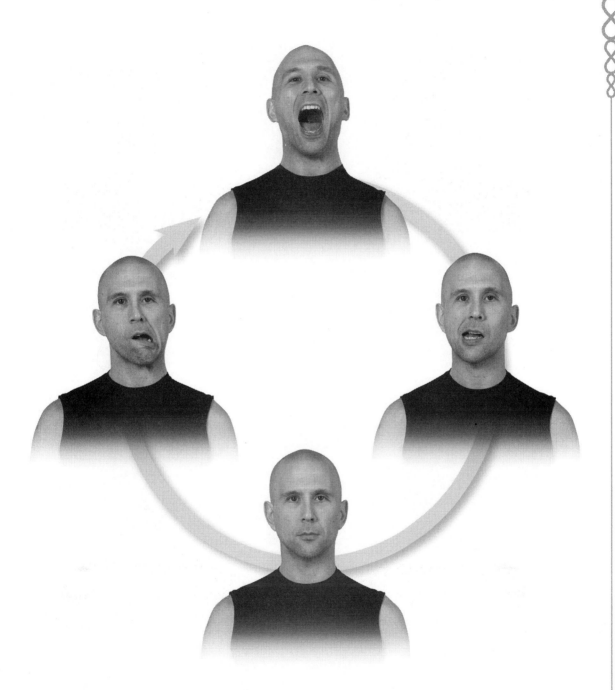

CIRCLES

Open – left – closed – right

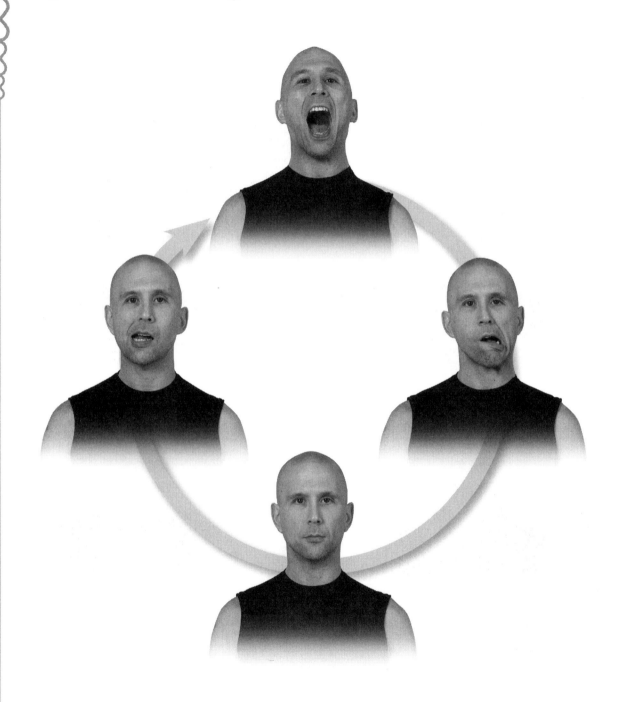

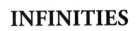

INFINITIES
Left – open – right – left – closed – right

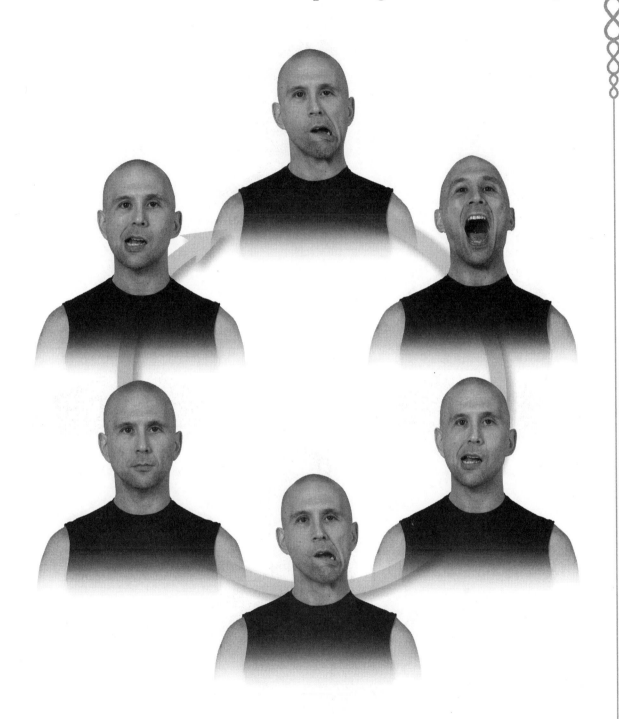

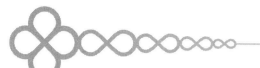

INFINITIES

Right – open – left – right – closed – left

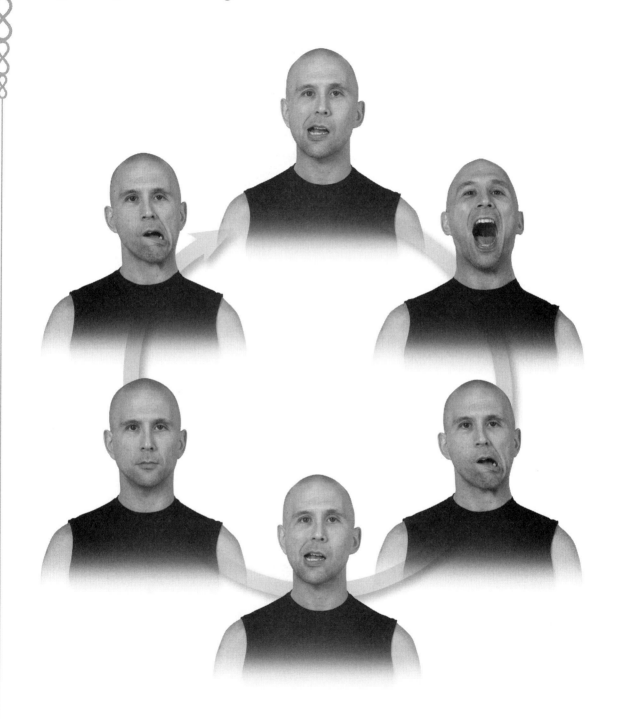

INFINITIES
Open – right – closed – open – left – closed

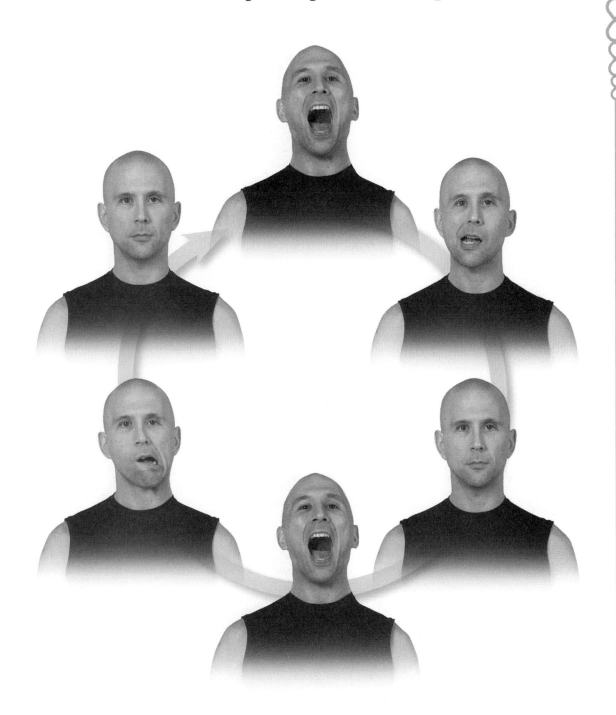

INFINITIES

Closed – right – open – closed – left – open

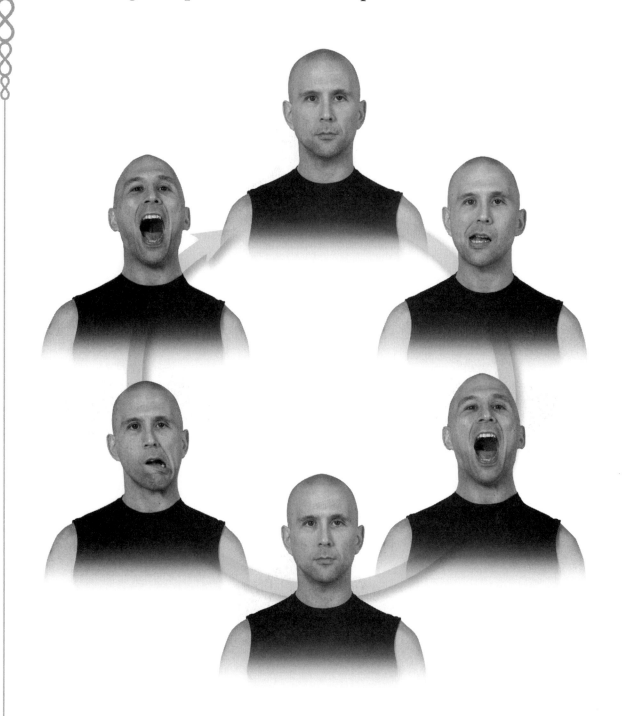

DIAGONAL INFINITIES
Open – right – left – closed – open

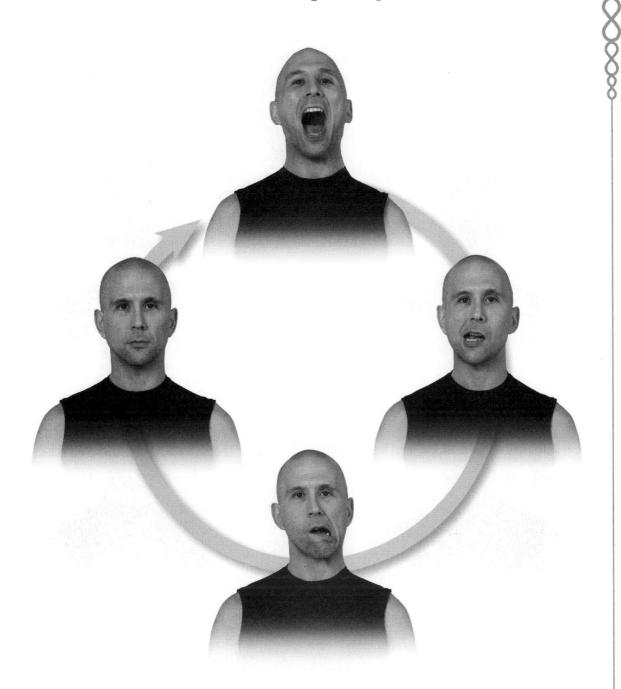

DIAGONAL INFINITIES

Closed – left – right – open – closed

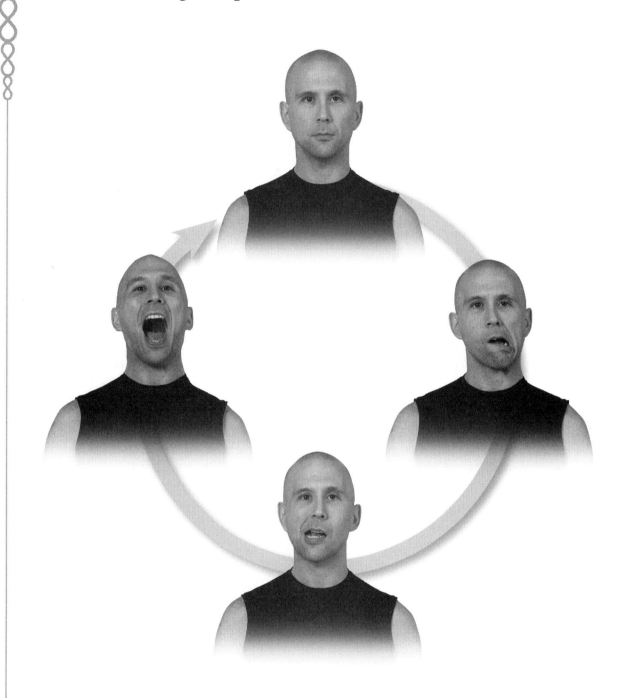

DIAGONAL INFINITIES
Open – left – right – closed – open

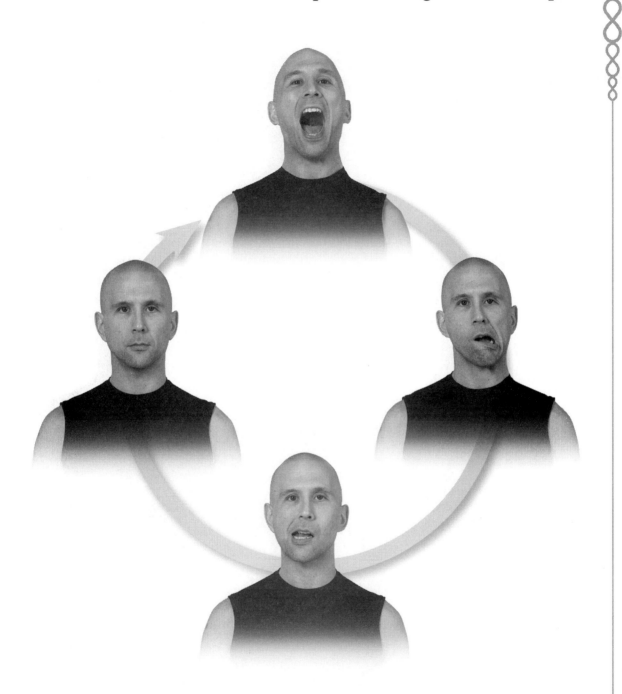

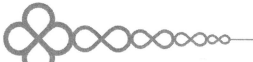

DIAGONAL INFINITIES
Closed – right – left – open – closed

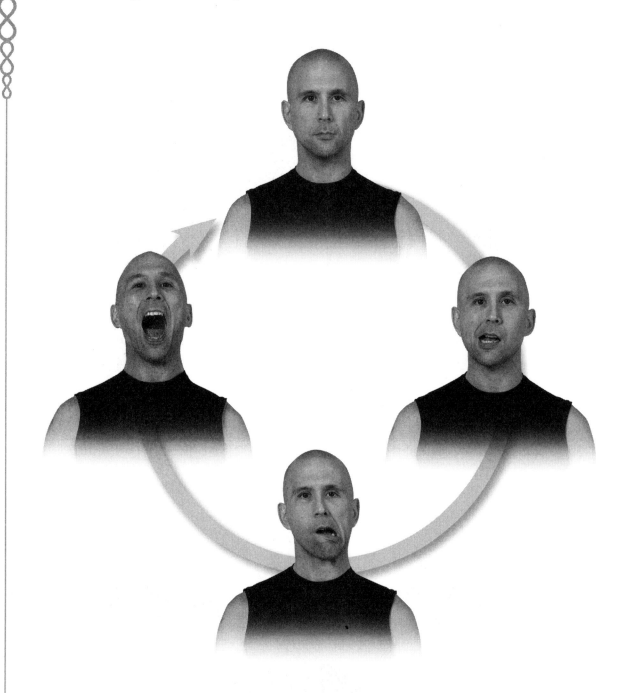

CLOVERS

Open – right – left – open – closed – left – right – closed

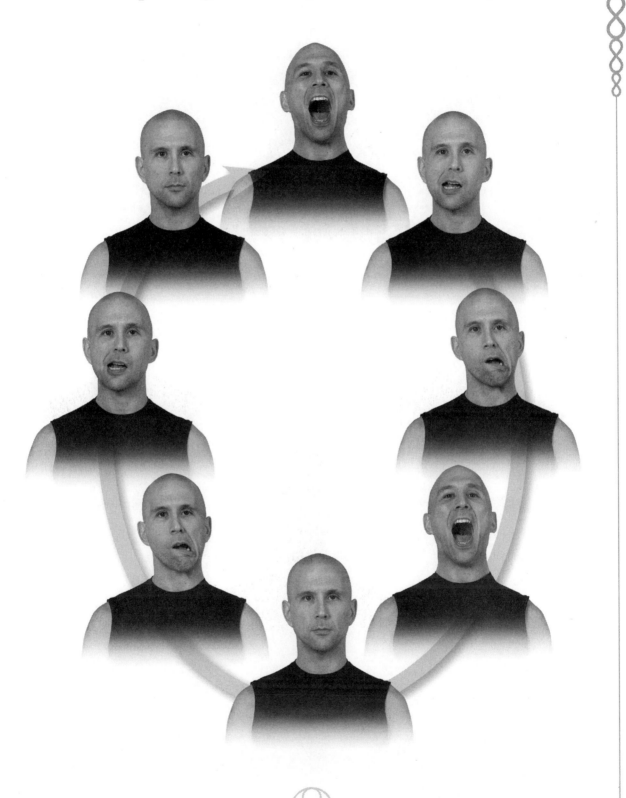

CLOVERS

Closed – right – left – closed – open – left – right – open

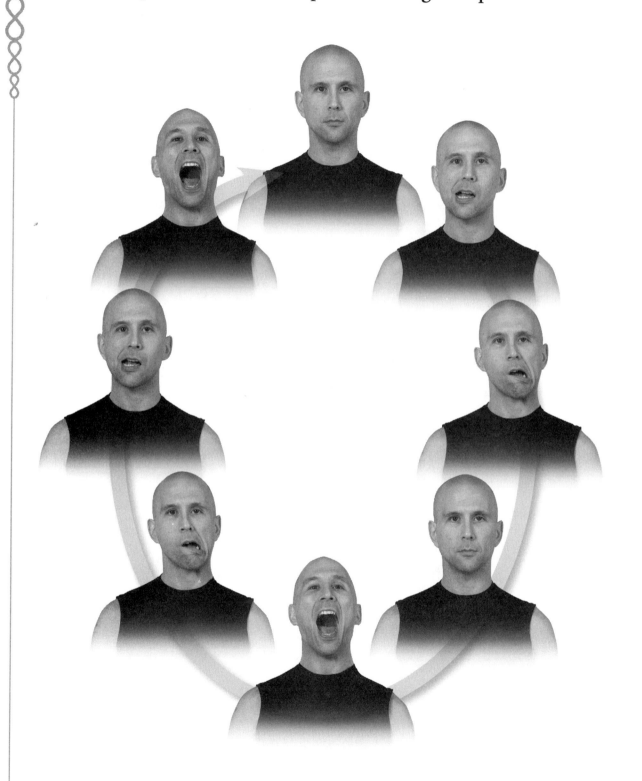

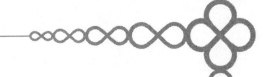

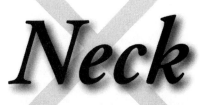

Neck

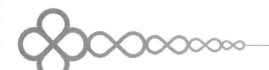

When not Free to Move from lack of prehabilitative movement due to stress, trauma, fear, overuse, underuse, or misuse, the following issues may result:

- Spasms
- Tight and tender
- Muscle strain
- Whiplash
- Neck stingers
- Torticollis
- Herniated disc
- Osteoarthritis

Common mental and emotional issues faced as a result of the area not being Free to Move:

- Not wanting to see others' points of view
- Trying to fix others
- Feeling like you've stuck your neck out
- Feeling like such and such is a pain in the neck
- Feeling like you want to wring his/her neck
- Feeling suffocated or strangled
- Fearing that you'll choke

Common organ referral affecting sensory-motor function of the area:

- The eyes (including visual problems) can refer pain to the back of the head and cause neck tightness.
- The thyroid gland can enlarge and alter motion of the neck.
- A dysfunctioning thyroid gland can also cause lower neck discomfort.
- Esophageal spasm (from something such as acid reflux) may cause some neck symptoms.
- Difficulty breathing may affect the lower muscles of the neck.

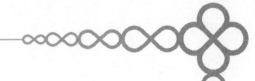

Neck mobility that will help you become Free to Move again:

1. **Ranges**
   a. Forward Glide
   b. Backward Glide
   c. Lateral Right
   d. Lateral Left
   e. Tilt Left
   f. Tilt Right
   g. Twist Left
   h. Twist Right
   i. Tilt Up
   j. Tilt Down

2. **Circles**
   a. Forward – right – backward – left
   b. Forward – left – backward – right

3. **Infinities**
   a. Left – forward – right – left – backward – right
   b. Right – forward – left – right – backward – left
   c. Forward – right – backward – forward – left – backward
   d. Backward – right – forward – backward – left – forward

4. **Diagonal infinities**
   a. Forward – right – left – backward – forward
   b. Backward – left – right – forward – backward
   c. Forward – left – right – backward – forward
   d. Backward – right – left – forward – backward

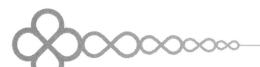

5. **Clovers**
   a. Forward – right – left – forward – backward – left
      – right – backward
   b. Backward – right – left – backward – forward – left
      – right – forward

6. **Waves**
   a. Jut chin – jaw right – tuck chin – jaw left
   b. Jut chin – jaw left – tuck chin – jaw right
   c. Drop atlas – tilt left – drop chin – tilt right
   d. Drop atlas – tilt right – drop chin – tilt left
   e. Tilt left – twist right – chin down – tilt right
      – twist left – chin down
   f. Tilt left – twist left – atlas back – tilt right
      – twist right – atlas back

RANGES

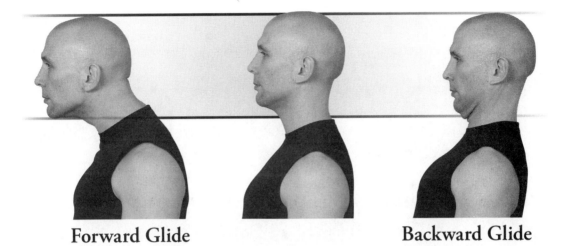

Forward Glide   Backward Glide

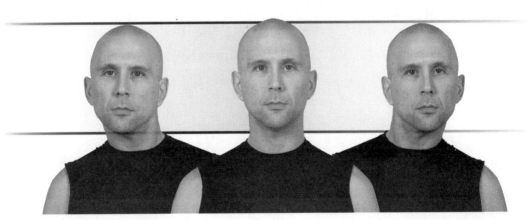

Lateral Right   Lateral Left

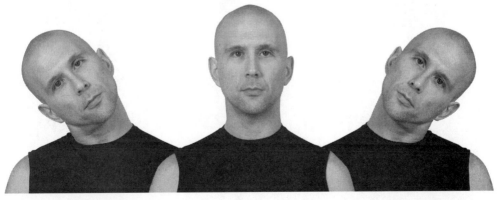

Tilt Right   Tilt Left

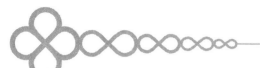

RANGES

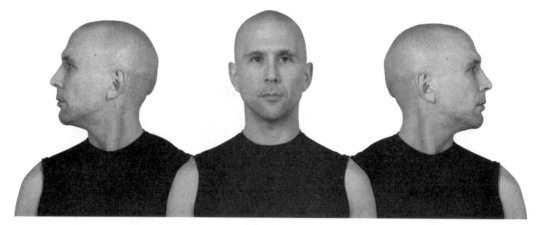

Twist Right   Twist Left

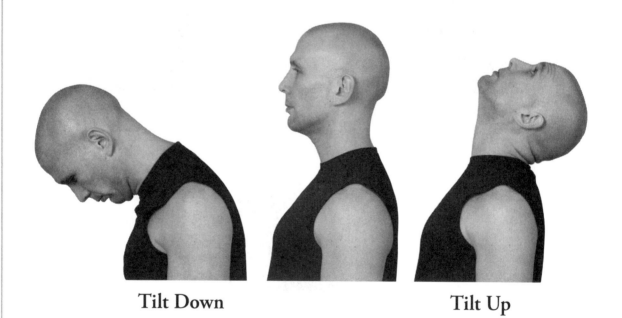

Tilt Down   Tilt Up

CIRCLES
Forward – right – backward – left
Forward – left – backward – right

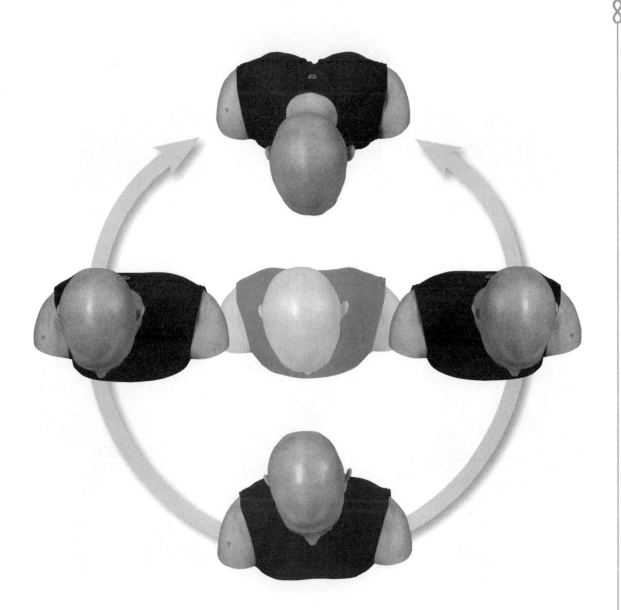

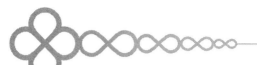

INFINITIES
Left – forward – right – left – backward – right

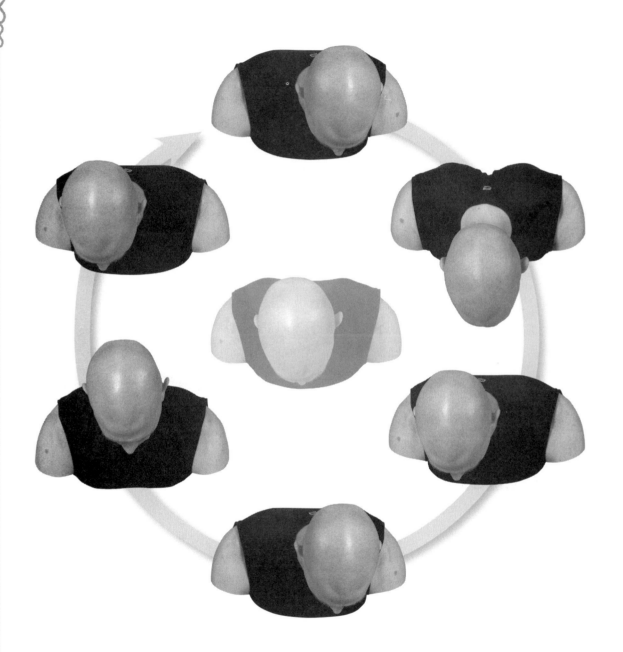

INFINITIES

Right – forward – left – right – backward – left

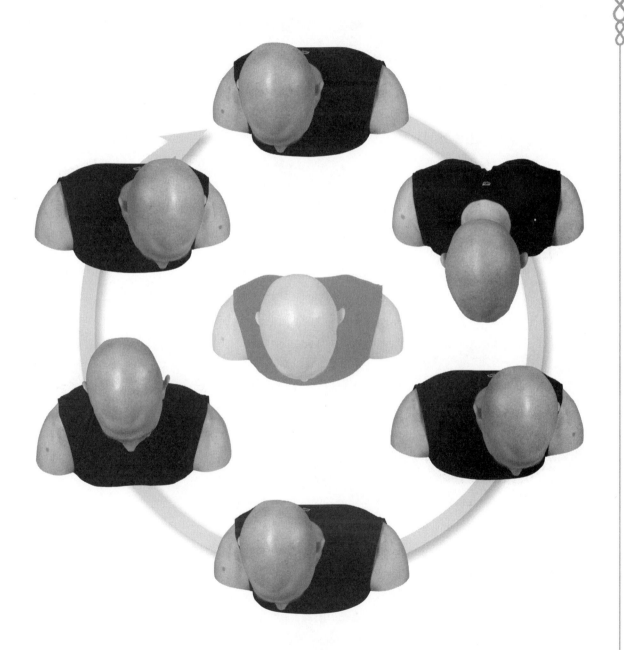

INFINITIES
Forward – right – backward – forward – left – backward

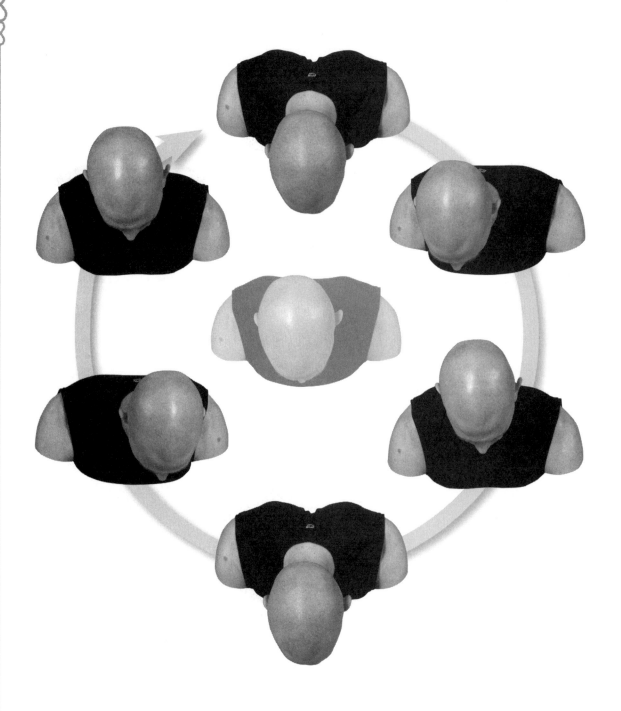

INFINITIES
Backward – right – forward – backward – left – forward

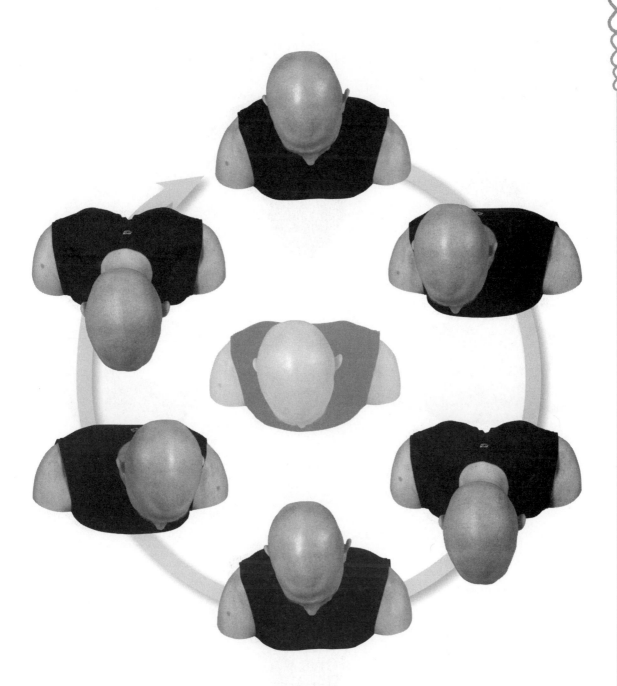

Free To Move

DIAGONAL INFINITIES
Forward – right – left – backward – forward

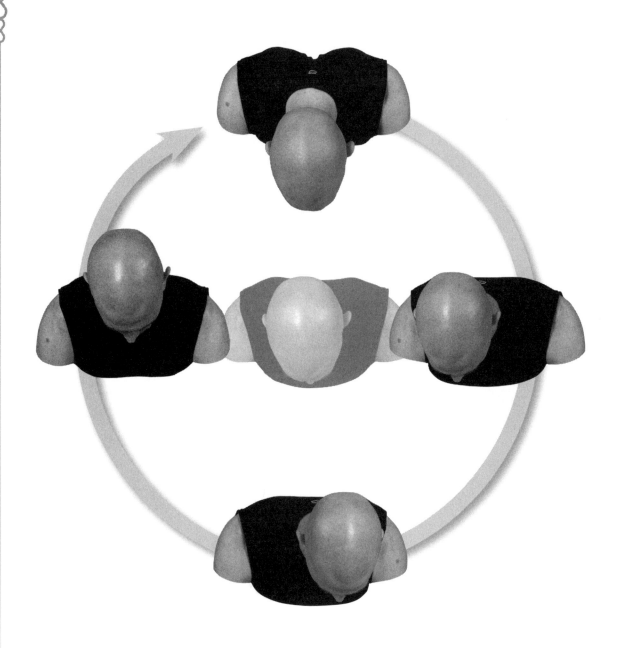

184

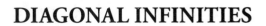

DIAGONAL INFINITIES
Backward – left – right – forward – backward

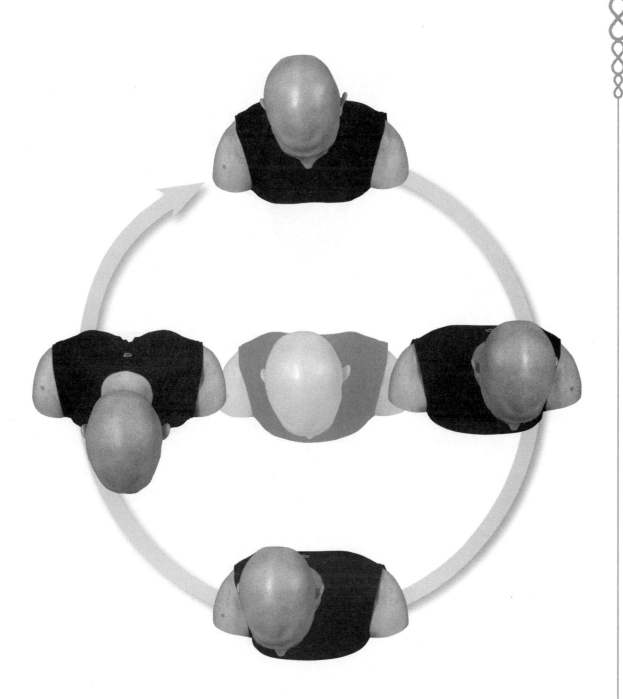

DIAGONAL INFINITIES

Forward – left – right – backward – forward

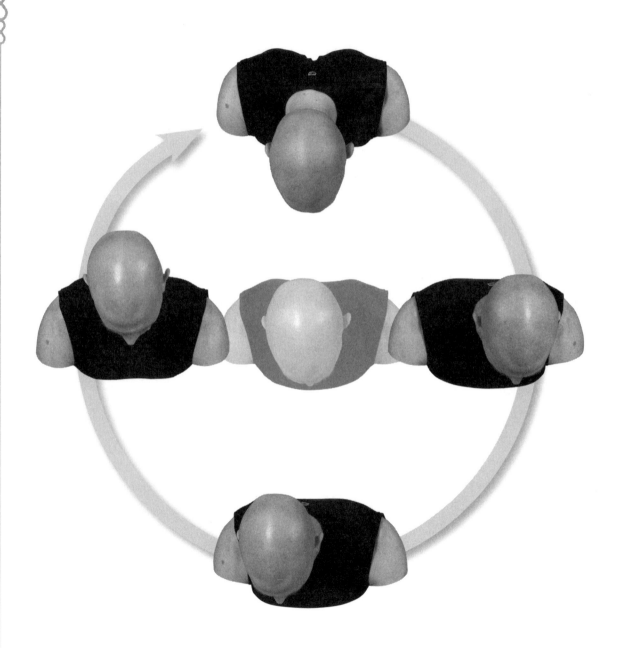

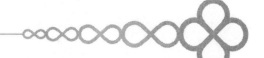

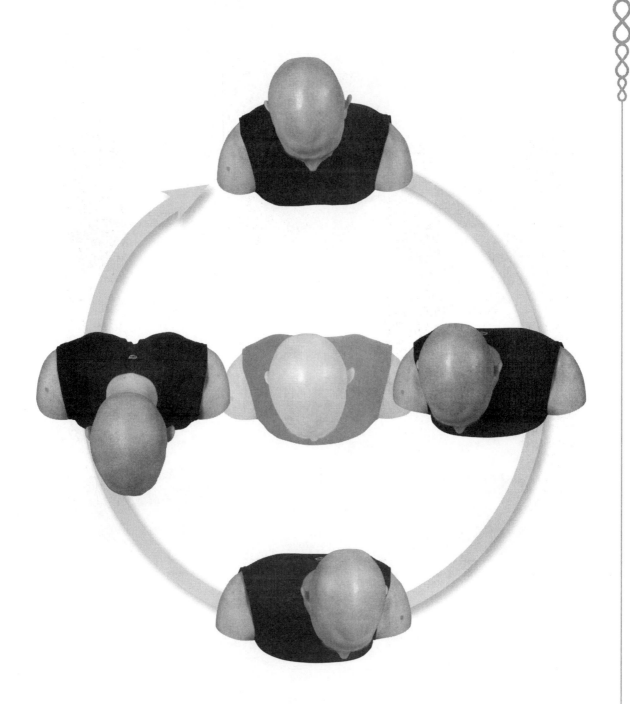

DIAGONAL INFINITIES
Backward – right – left – forward – backward

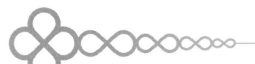

CLOVERS

Forward – right – left – forward – backward – left – right – backward

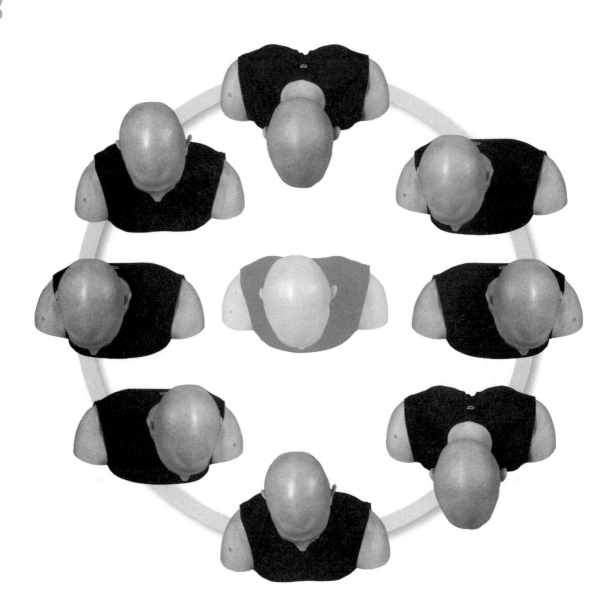

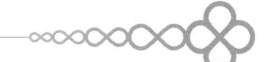

CLOVERS

Backward – right – left – backward – forward – left – right – forward

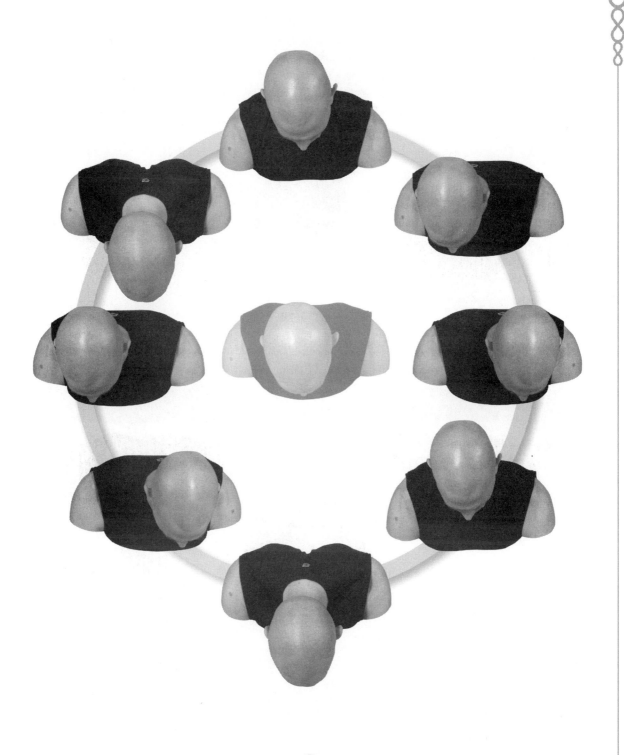

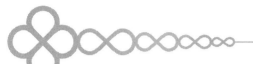

WAVES

Jut chin – jaw right – tuck chin – jaw left

Jut chin – jaw left – tuck chin – jaw right

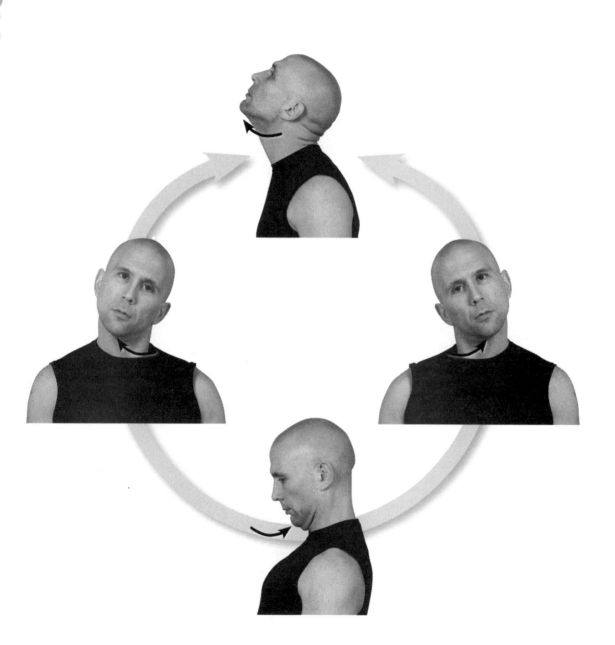

WAVES

Drop atlas – tilt left – drop chin – tilt right

Drop atlas – tilt right – drop chin – tilt left

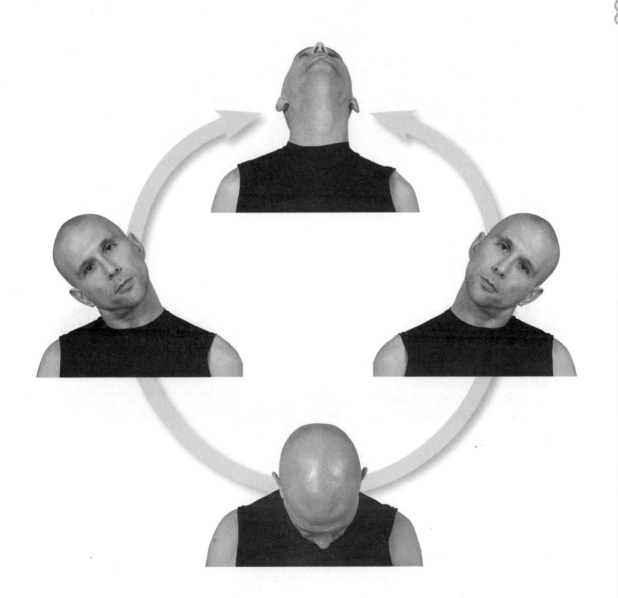

WAVES

Tilt left – twist right – chin down – tilt right – twist left – chin down

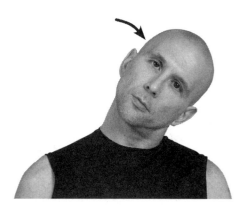
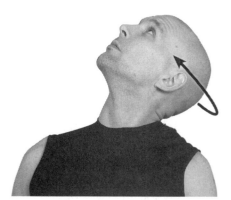

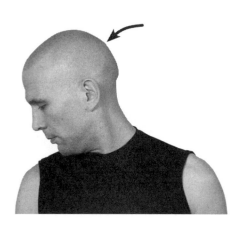
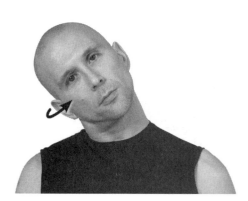

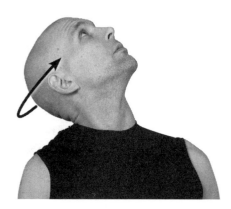
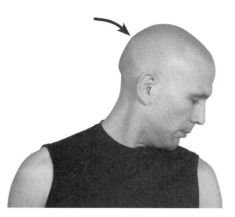

WAVES

Tilt left – twist left – atlas back – tilt right – twist right – atlas back

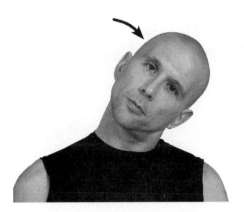
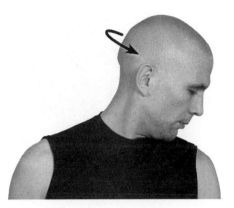

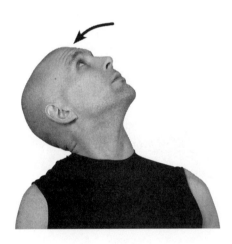
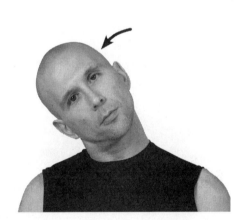

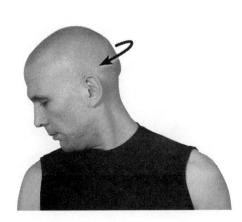
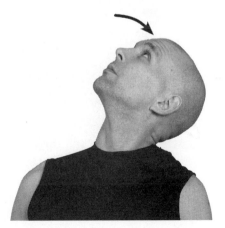

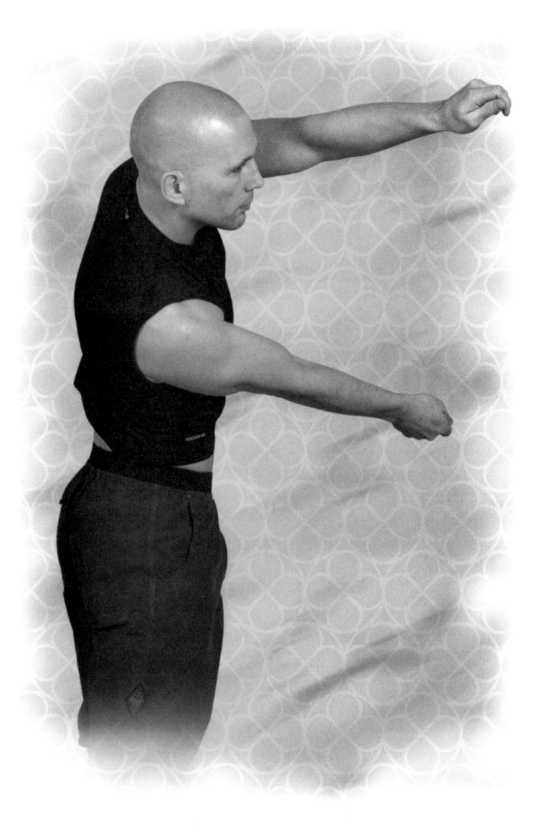

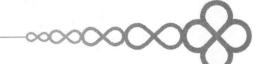

Shoulders

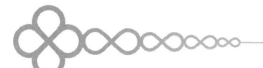

When not Free to Move from lack of prehabilitative movement due to stress, trauma, fear, overuse, underuse, or misuse, the following issues may result:

- Rotator cuff impingement
- Tendonitis
- Sternoclavicular joint dislocation
- Acromioclavicular joint separation
- Dislocation and subluxation
- Osteoarthritis
- Bursitis

Common mental and emotional issues faced as a result of area not being Free to Move:

- We carry our experiences and their emotions here
- Feeling that life is a heavy burden
- Sometimes shouldering too much responsibility is possible
- Feeling that we don't have a shoulder to cry on

Common organ referral affecting sensory-motor function of the area:

- The heart can refer pain most commonly to the left shoulder, but in some instances the right shoulder is also involved.
- The liver can refer pain to the right shoulder.
- The diaphragm can refer to either shoulder.
- If there is pancreatic inflammation or disease, pain or discomfort can be referred to the left shoulder indirectly through irritation of the left diaphragm.
- The gallbladder can refer pain to the right scapular (shoulder blade) region.
- Sometimes the lungs refer pain to the shoulders.
- While it is not technically organ referral, sometimes a neck problem (such as a herniated disc in the neck or a nerve entrapment syndrome) can cause shoulder pain.

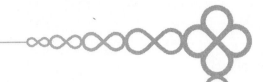

Shoulder mobility that will help you become Free to Move again:

7. **Ranges**
   a. Steeple
   b. Handcuff
   c. Rear Trigger
   d. Overhead Trigger
   e. Arm Screw

8. **Circles**
   a. Overhead Clockwise (CW)
   b. Overhead Counter-Clockwise (CCW)
   c. Outside Clockwise
   d. Outside Counter-Clockwise
   e. Inside Clockwise
   f. Inside Counter-Clockwise
   g. Bottom Clockwise
   h. Bottom Counter-Clockwise
   i. Front Clockwise
   j. Front Counter-Clockwise
   k. Back Clockwise
   l. Back Counter-Clockwise
   m. Camshaft Rear
   n. Camshaft Front

9. **Infinities**
   a. Inside – Outside
   b. Outside – Inside
   c. Top – Bottom
   d. Bottom – Top
   e. Front – Back
   f. Back – Front

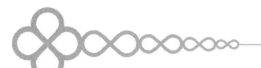

10. **Clovers**
    a. Front – inside – outside – top – bottom – back

11. **Waves**
    a. Alternating Double Infinities Dropping (Hammers)
    b. Alternating Double Infinities Swimming

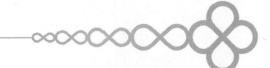

Steeple

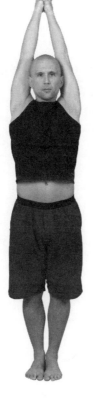

Handcuff

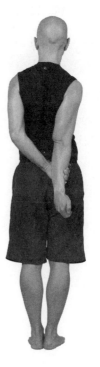

Rear Trigger

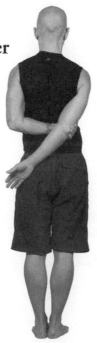

Overhead Trigger

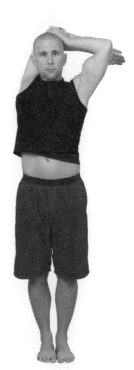

RANGES

Arm Screw

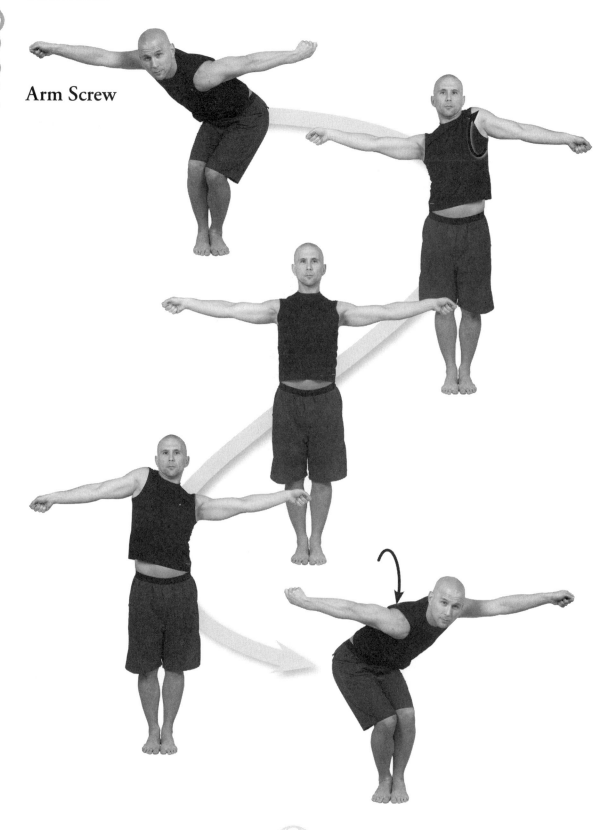

Arm Screw
(continued)

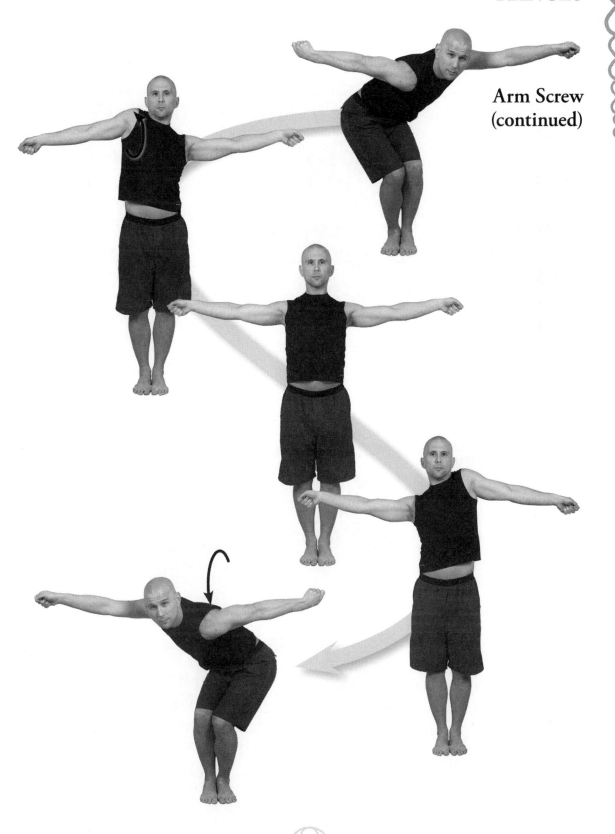

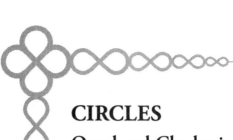

CIRCLES
Overhead Clockwise

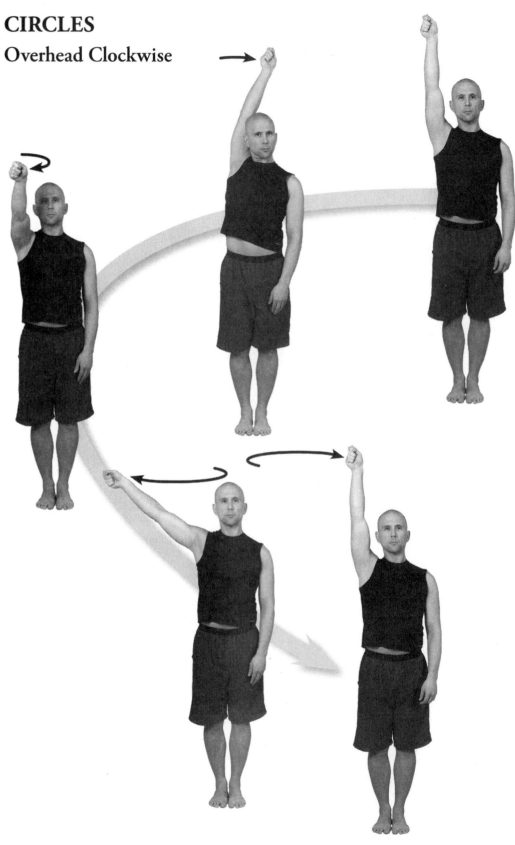

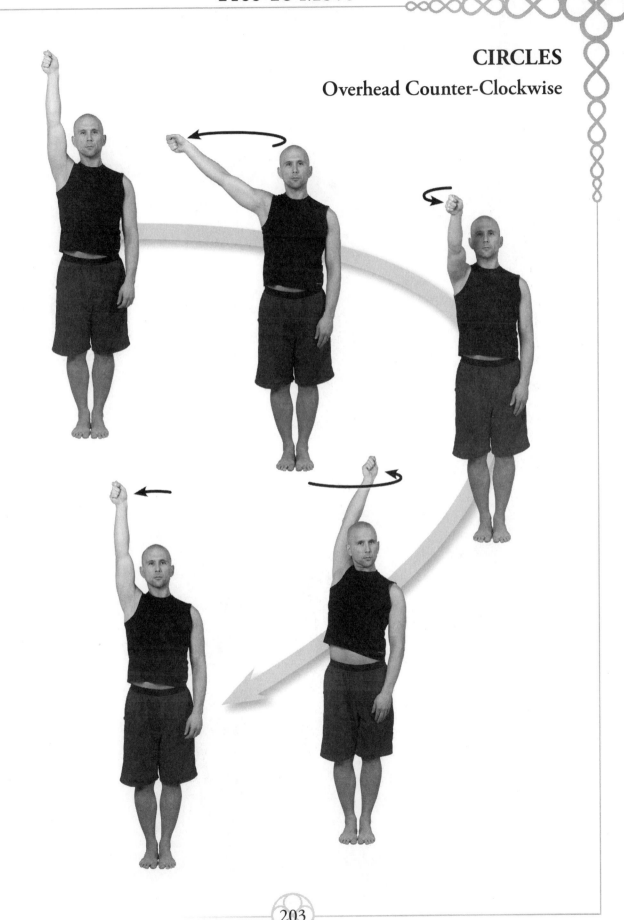

CIRCLES
Outside Backward

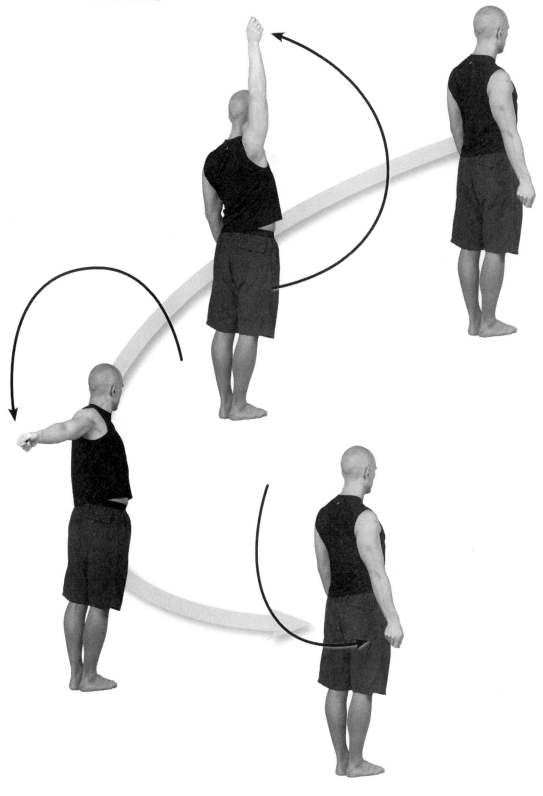

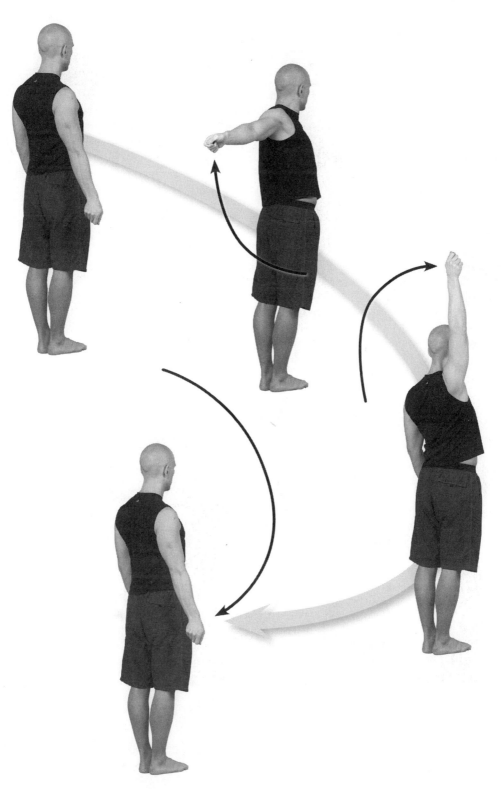

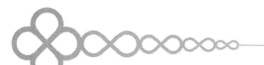

CIRCLES
Inside Clockwise

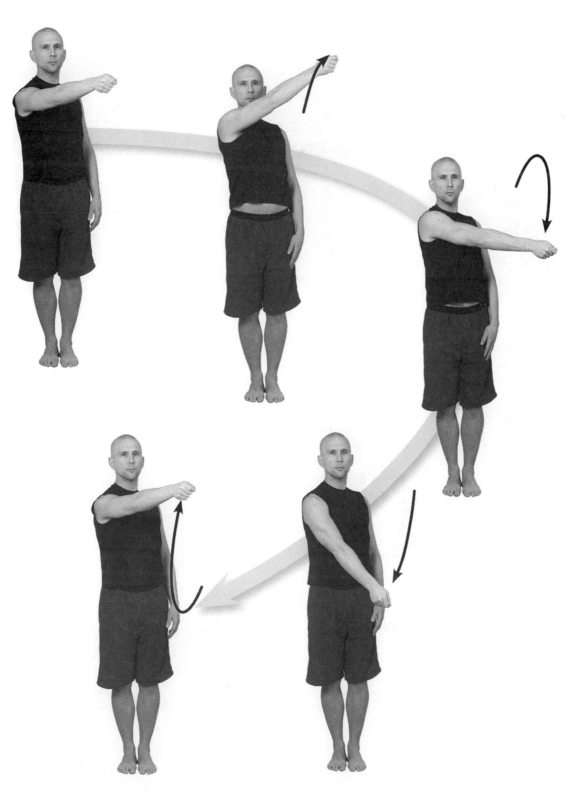

CIRCLES
Bottom Clockwise

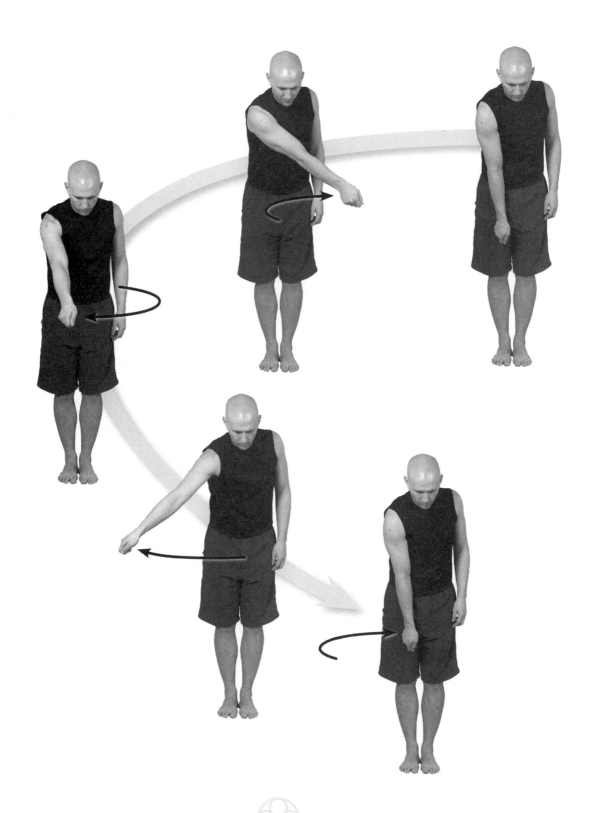

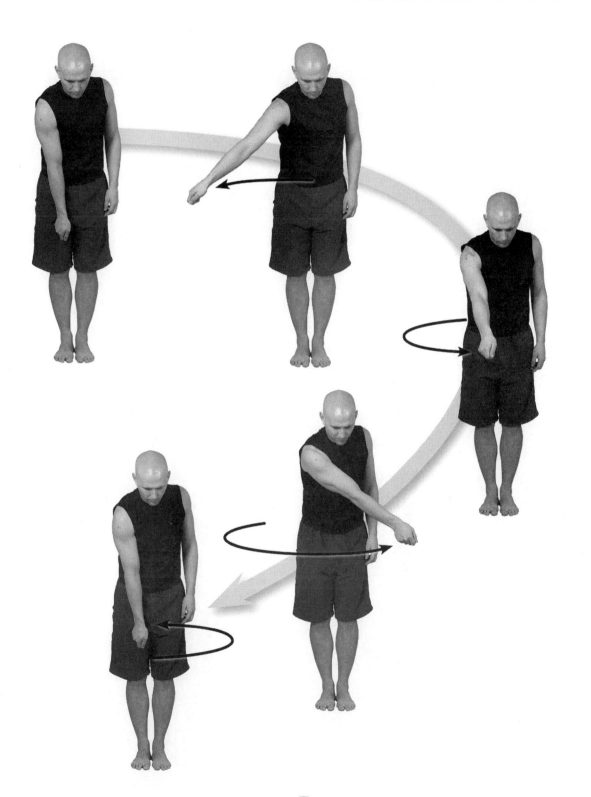

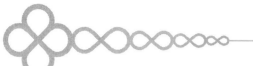

CIRCLES
Front Clockwise

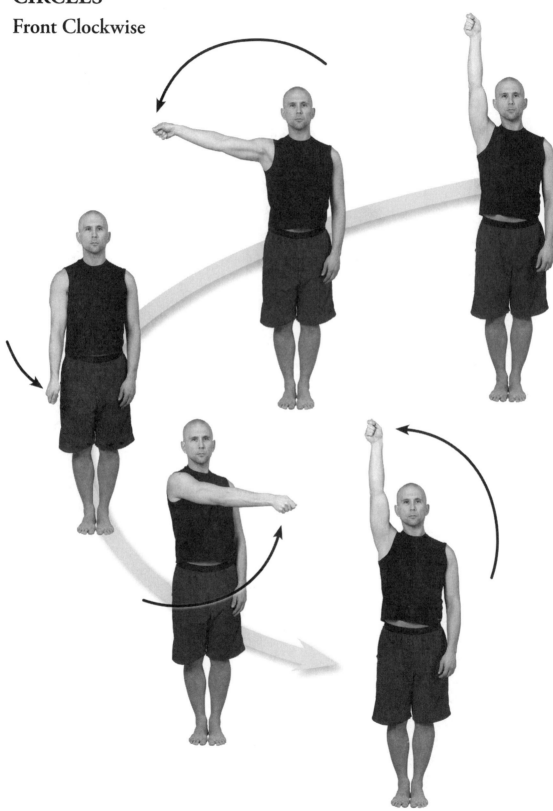

CIRCLES
Front Counter-Clockwise

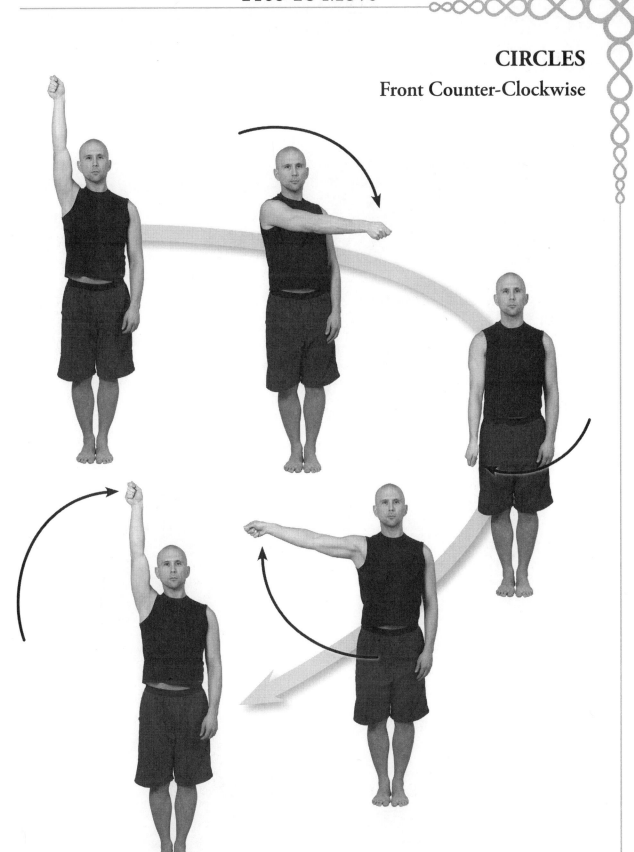

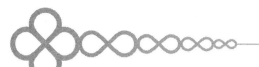

CIRCLES

Back Clockwise

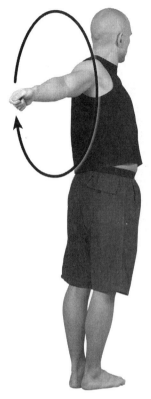

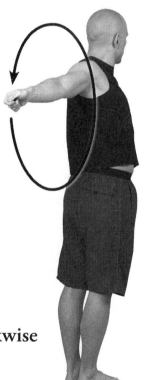

Back Counter-Clockwise

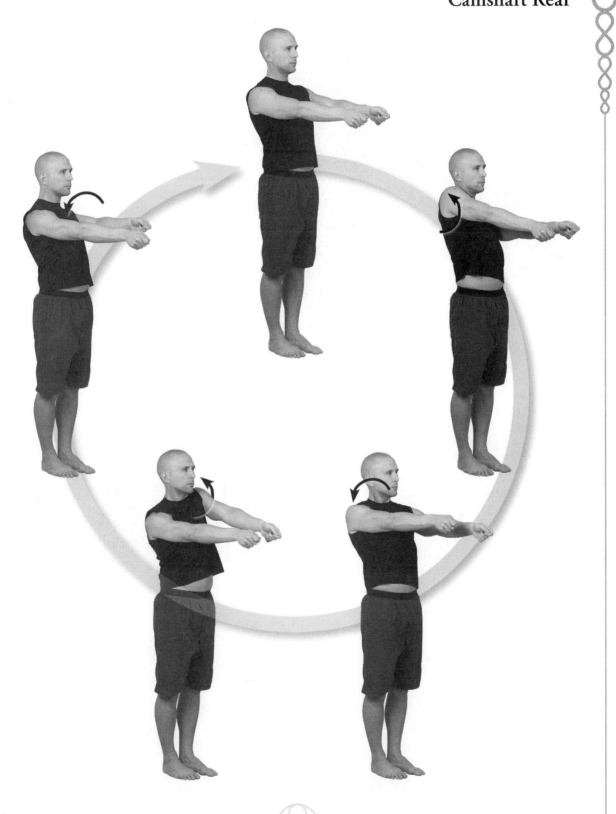

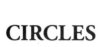

CIRCLES
Camshaft Front

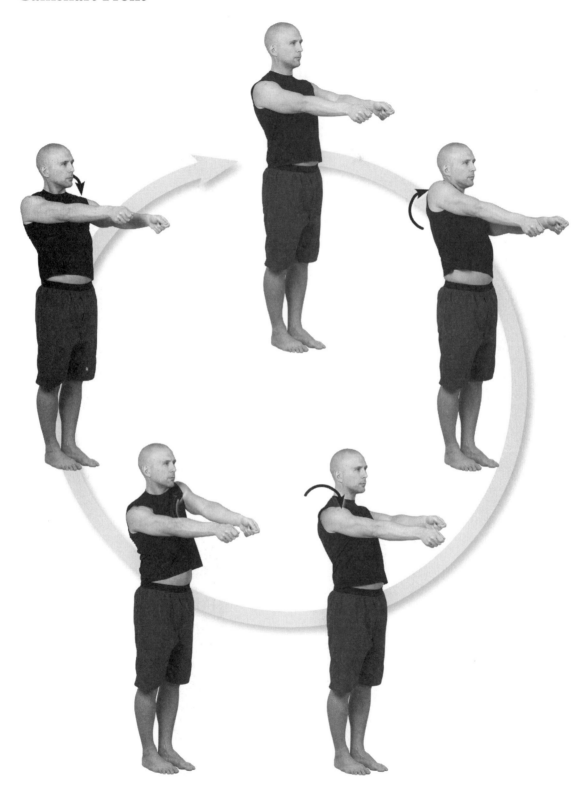

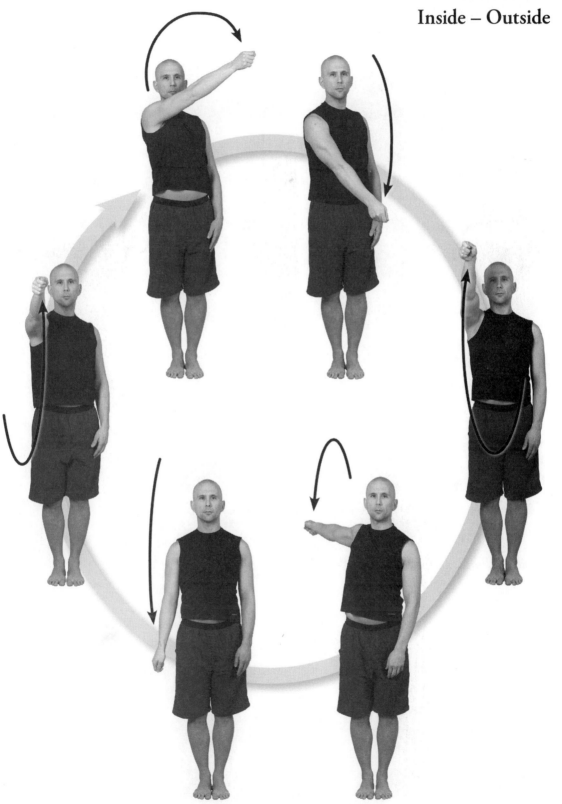

INFINITIES
Outside – Inside

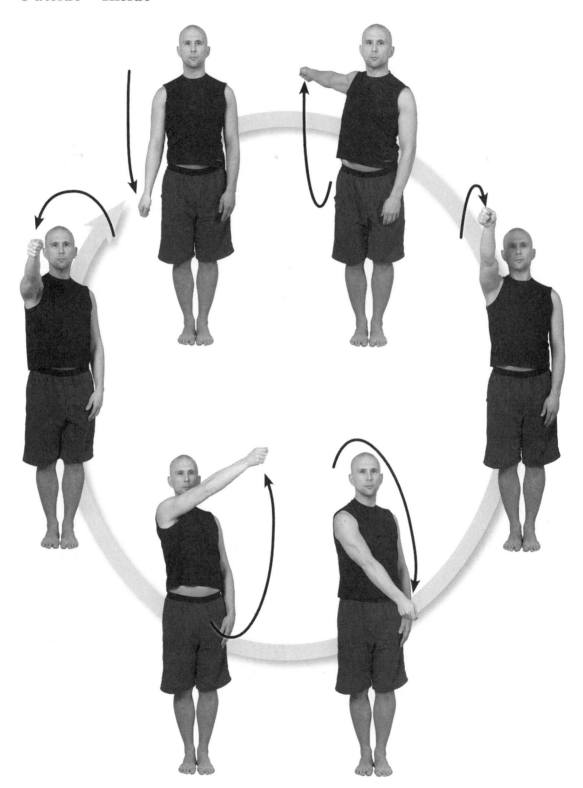

INFINITIES
Top – Bottom

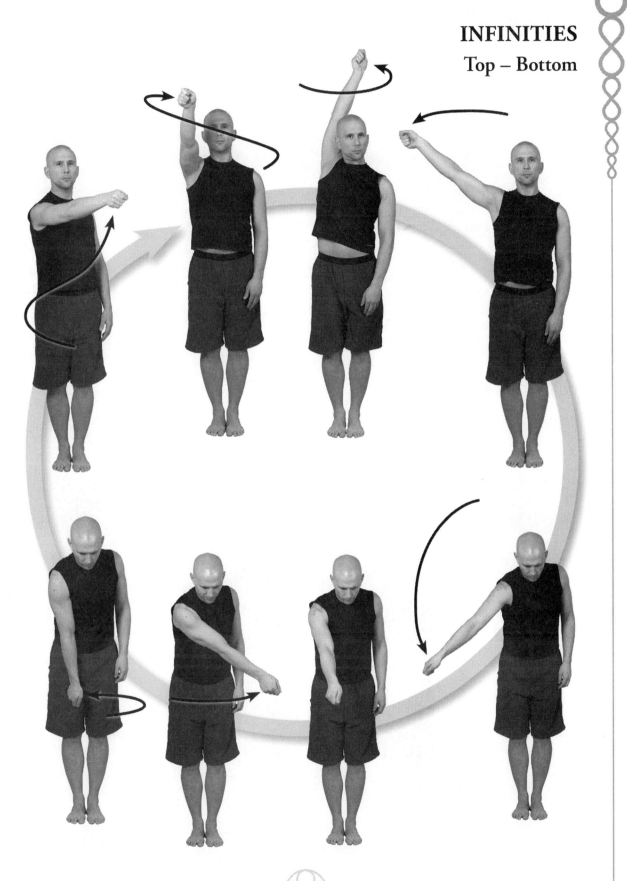

INFINITIES
Bottom – Top

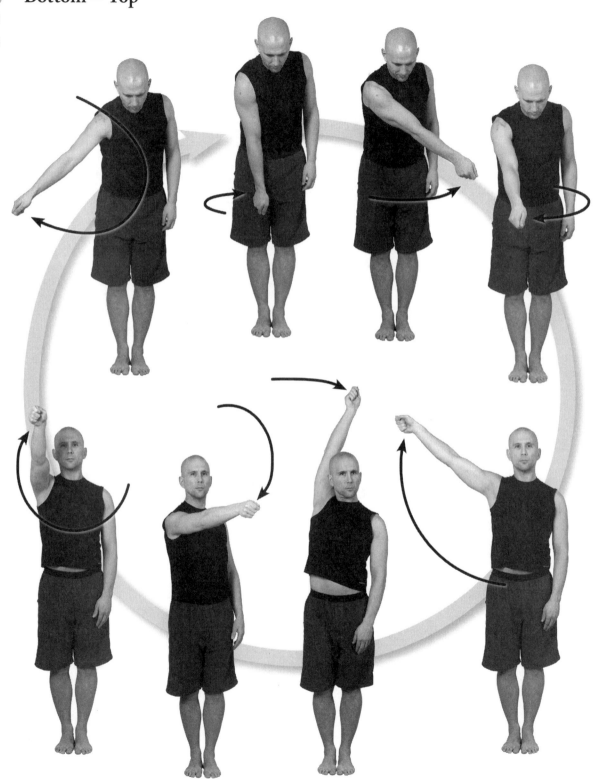

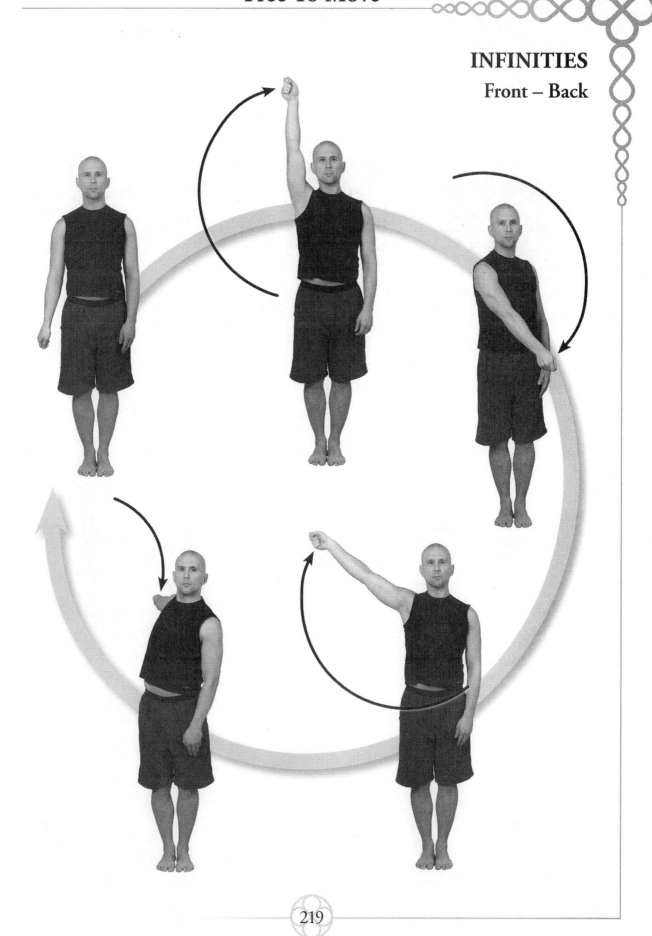

INFINITIES
Back – Front

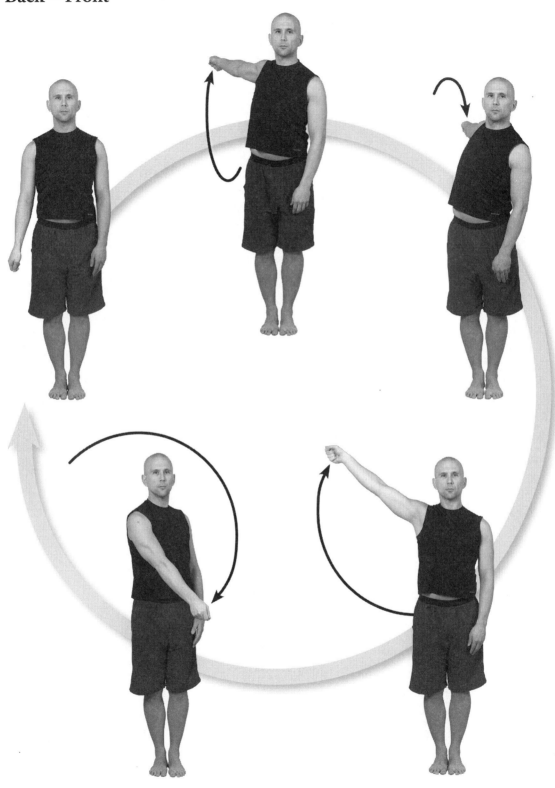

CLOVERS
Front – inside – outside – top – bottom – back

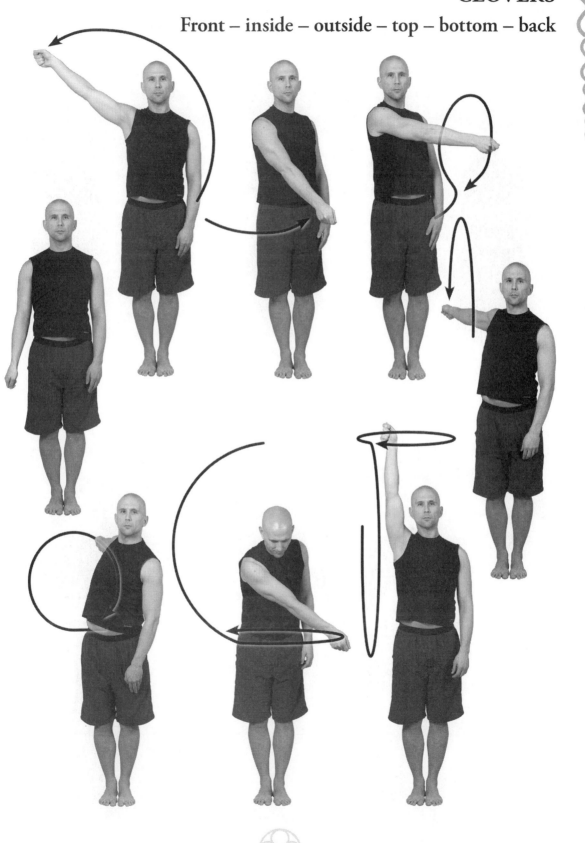

WAVES

Alternating Double Infinities Dropping Hammers

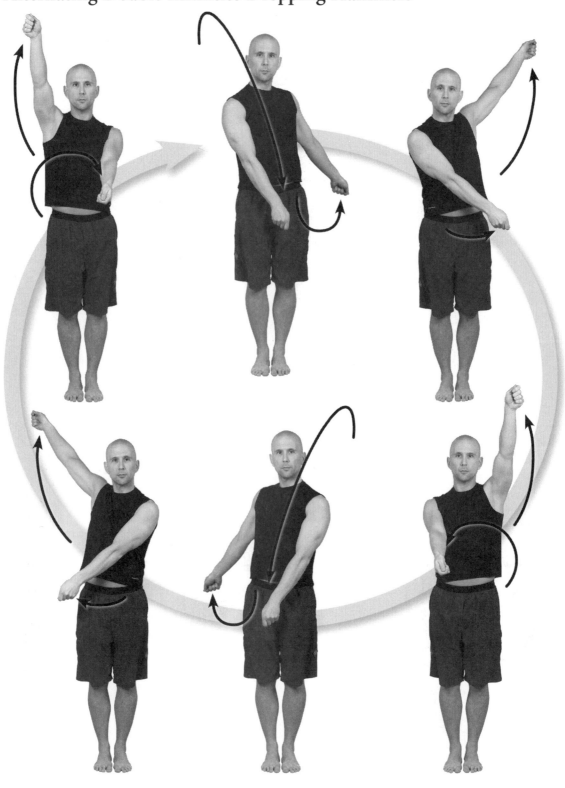

WAVES
Alternating Double Infinities Swimming

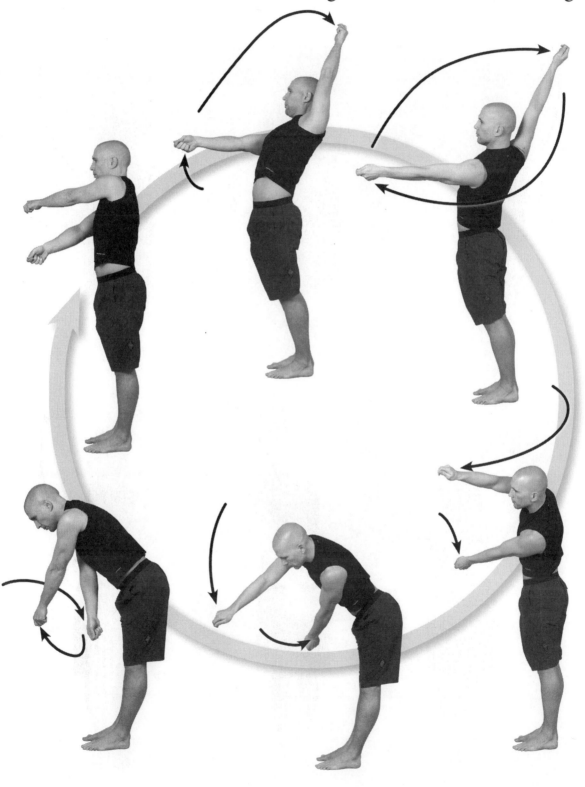

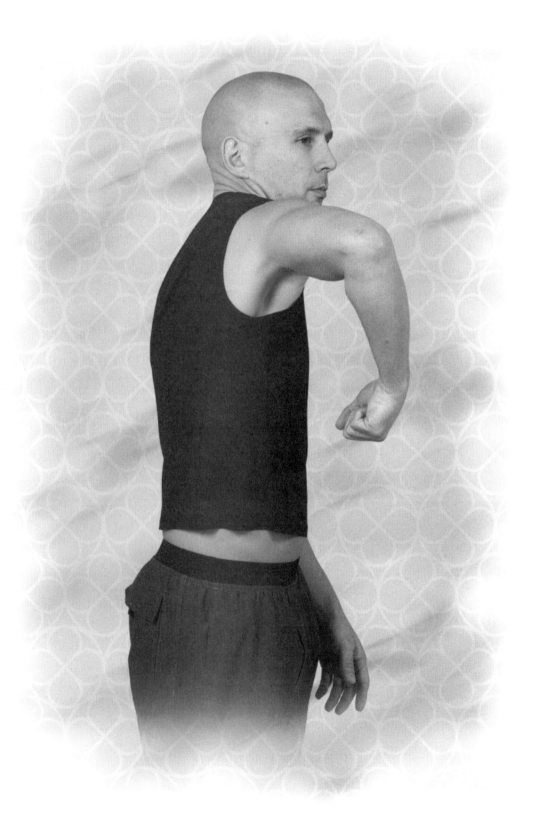

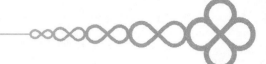

Elbows

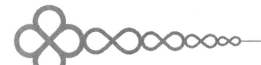

When not Free to Move from lack of prehabilitative movement due to stress, trauma, fear, overuse, underuse, or misuse, the following issues may result:

- Lateral epicondylitis, also referred to as tennis elbow
- Medial epicondylitis, also referred to as golfer's elbow
- Osteoarthritis

Common mental and emotional issues faced as a result of area not being Free to Move:

- We are clutching too much, too strongly for too long.
- We are pushing too hard.
- We can feel that we can't hold on to life.
- We can experience the intense monotony of repeating the same thing everyday.

Common organ referral affecting sensory-motor function of the area:

- There are no organs that refer pain directly to the elbow.
- While it is not technically organ referral, sometimes a neck problem (such as a herniated disc in the neck or a nerve entrapment syndrome) can cause elbow pain.

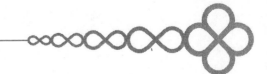

Elbow mobility that will help you become Free to Move again:

12. **Ranges**
    a. Flag
    b. Steeple
    c. Hitch Hiker
    d. Thumbs Down

13. **Circles**
    a. Hitch Hiker
    b. Butter Churn
    c. Outside
    d. Speed Bag

14. **Infinity**
    a. Top – Bottom
    b. Bottom – Top
    c. Front – Back
    d. Back – Front
    e. Right – Left
    f. Left – Right

15. **Clovers**
    a. Top – bottom – right – left

16. **Waves**
    a. Elbow Cam Inside
    b. Elbow Cam Outside
    c. Shoulder – elbow – wrist
    d. Wrist – elbow – shoulder

RANGES

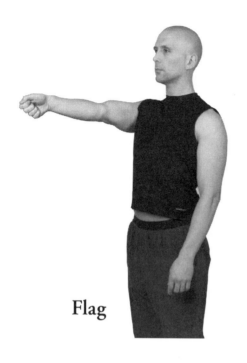

Flag

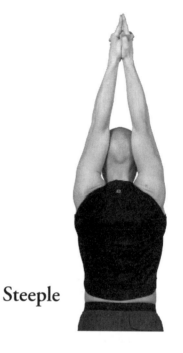

Steeple

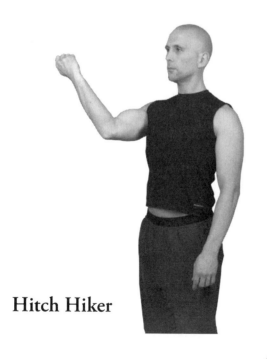

Hitch Hiker

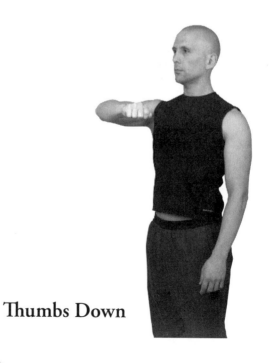

Thumbs Down

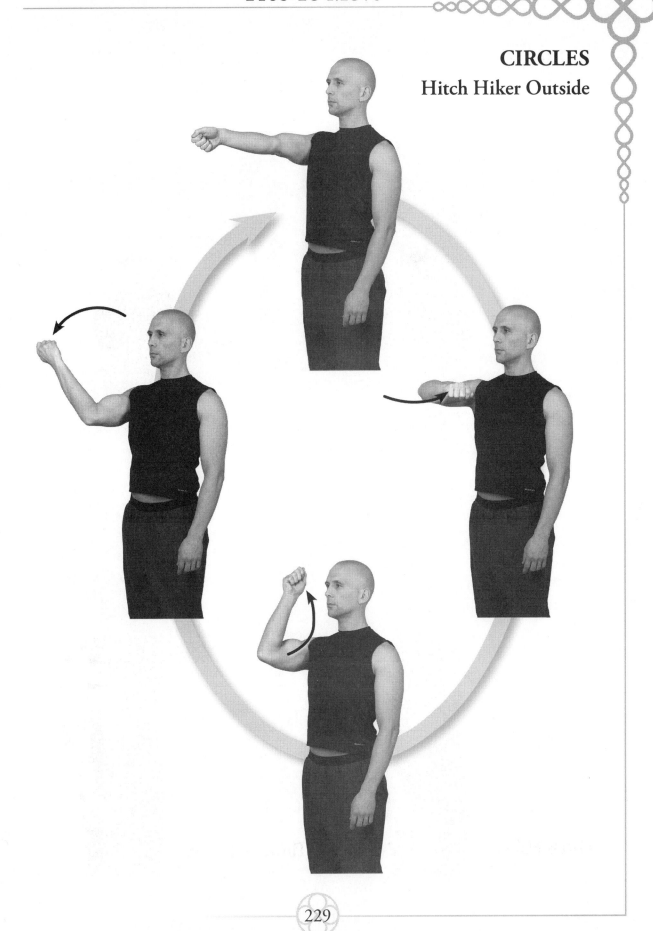

CIRCLES
Hitch Hiker Inside

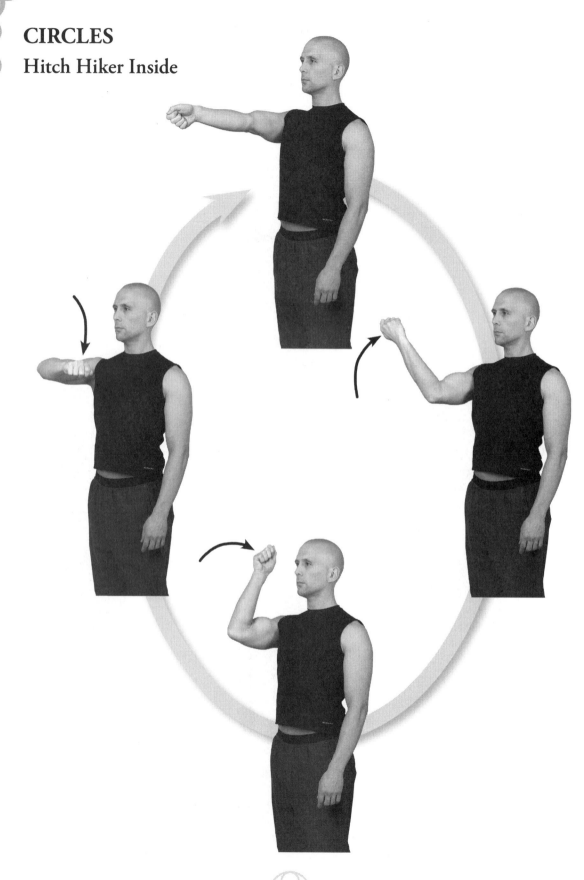

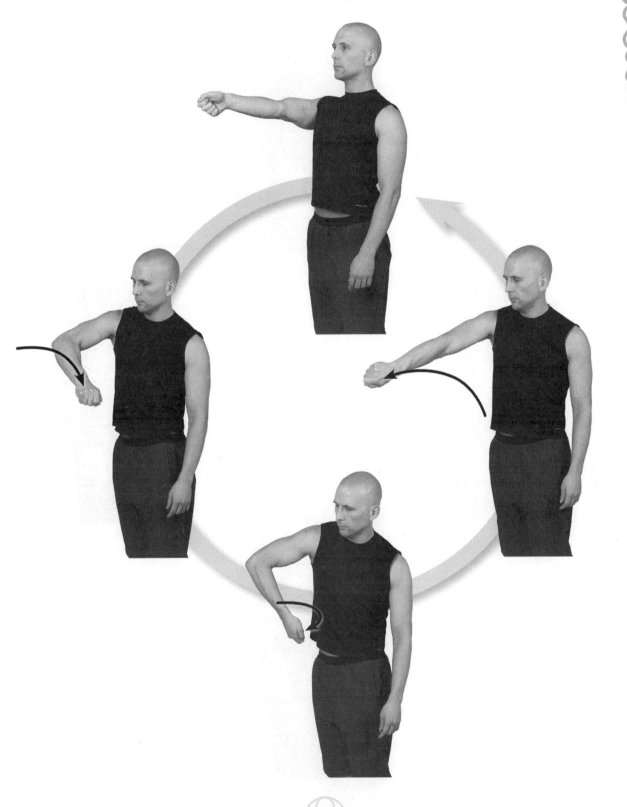

CIRCLES
Butter Churn Clockwise

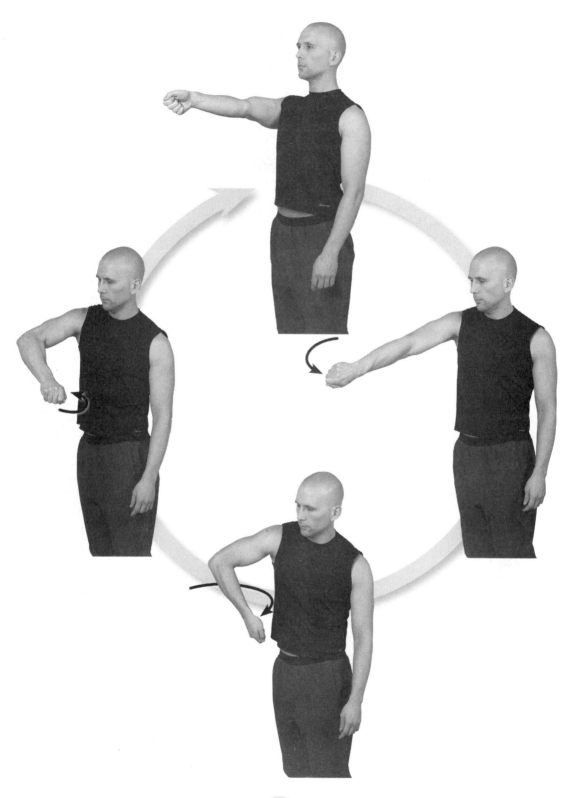

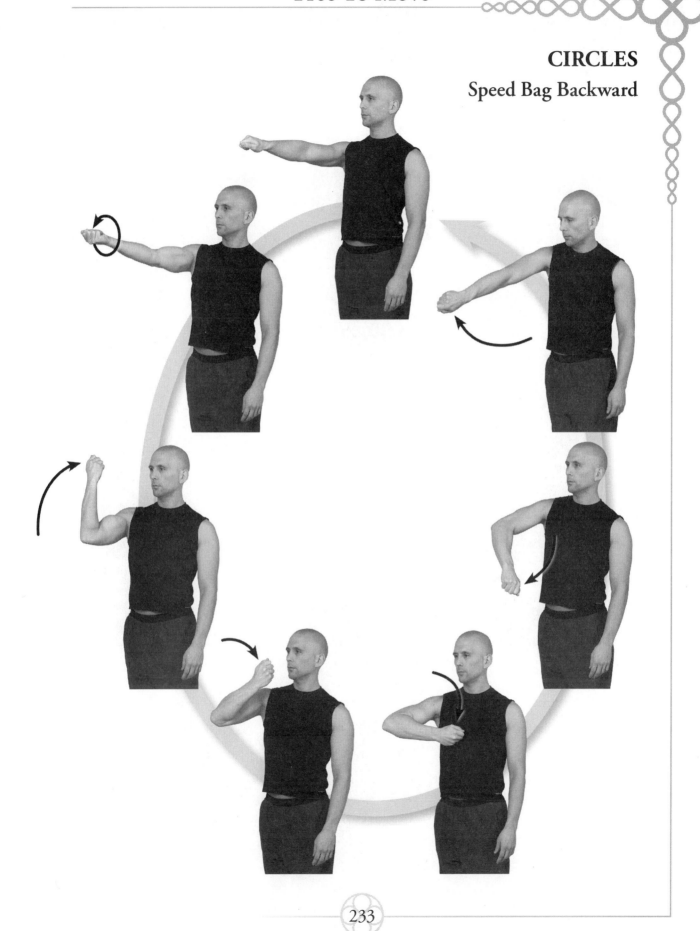

CIRCLES
Speed Bag Forward

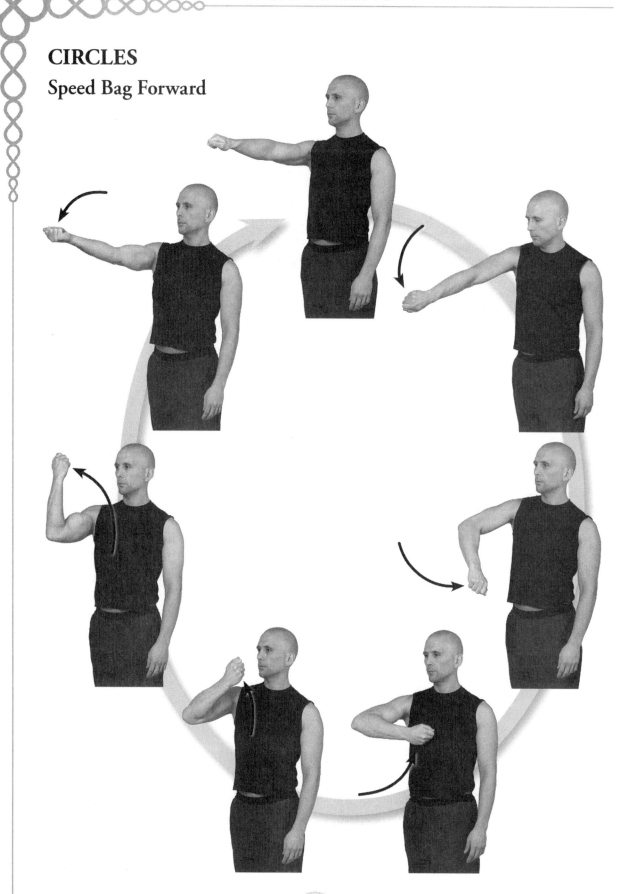

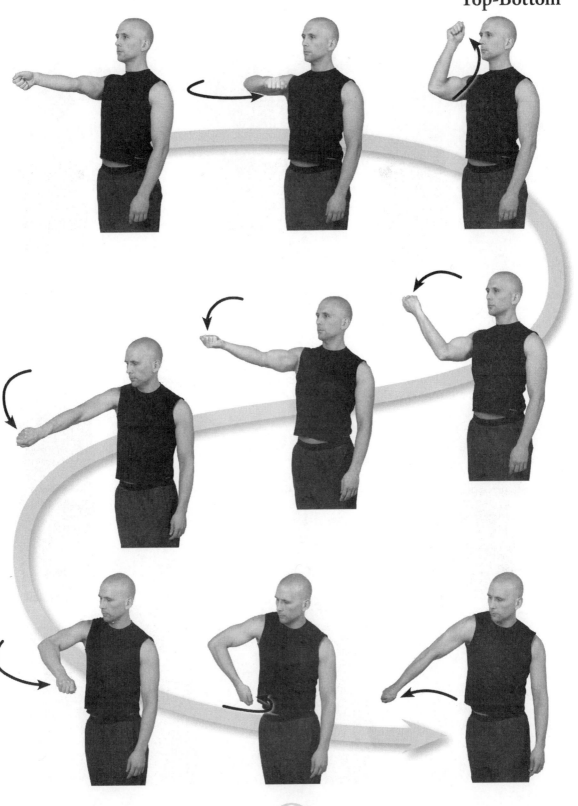

INFINITIES
Bottom-Top

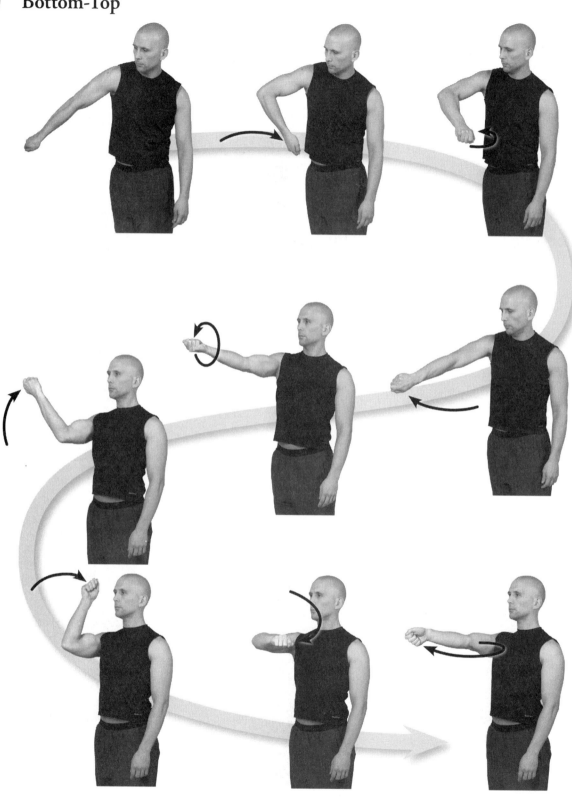

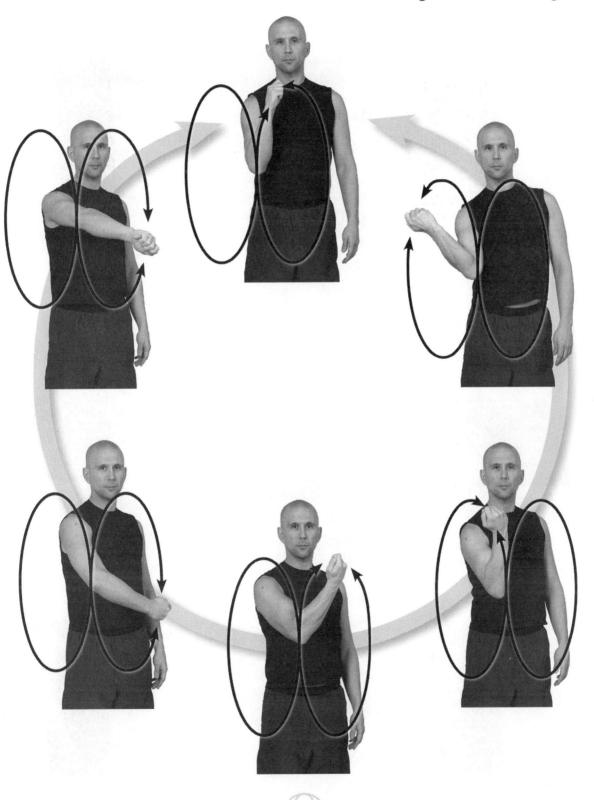

CLOVERS
Top – bottom – right – left

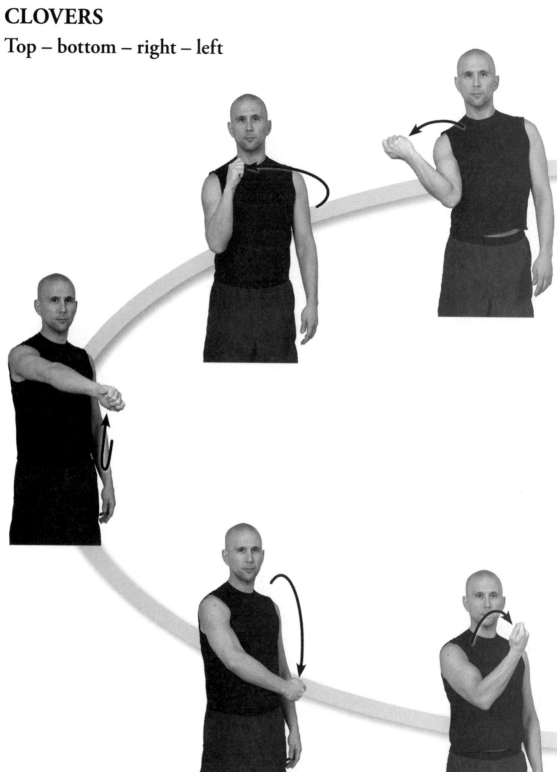

CLOVERS
Top – bottom – right – left

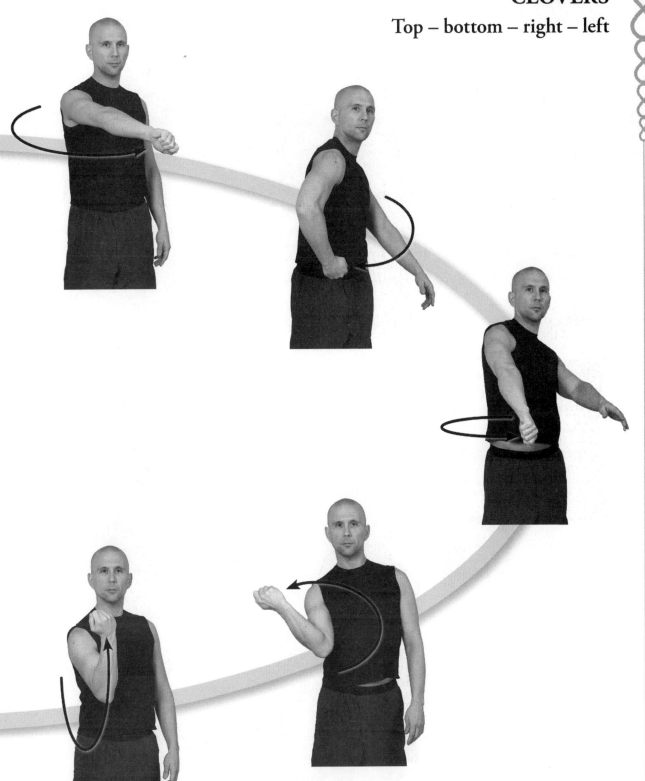

WAVES
Elbow Cam Inside

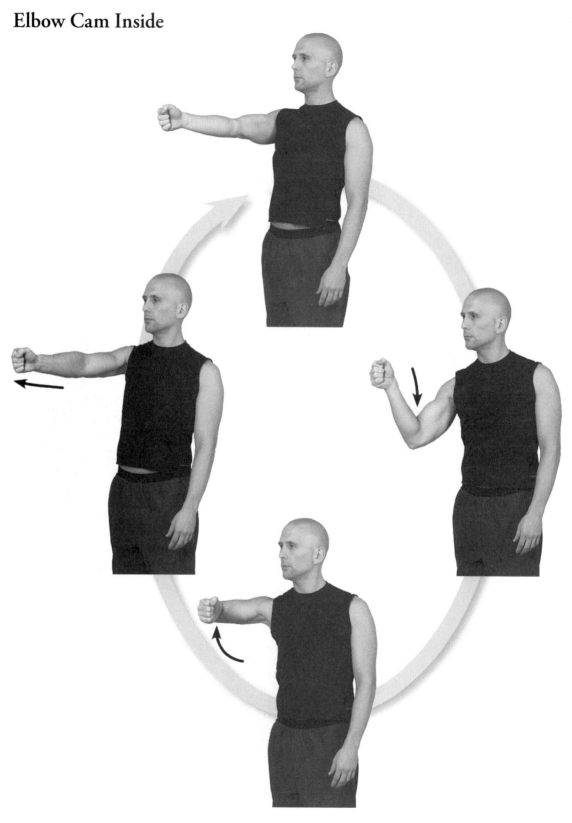

WAVES
Elbow Cam Outside

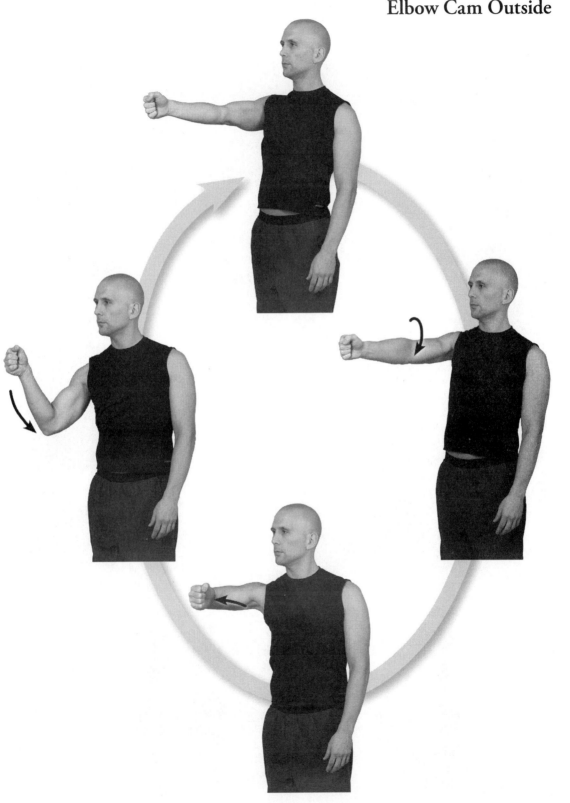

WAVES

Shoulder – elbow – wrist

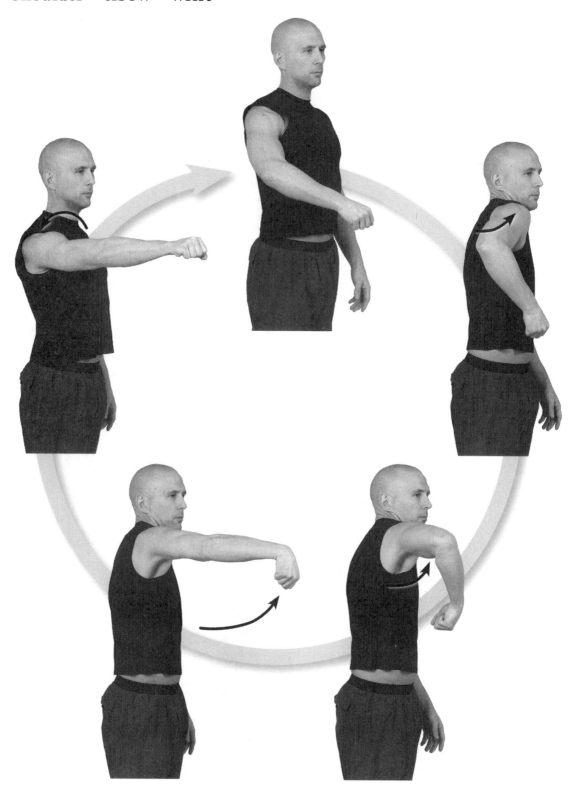

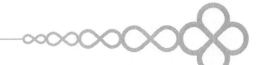

WAVES
Wrist – elbow – shoulder

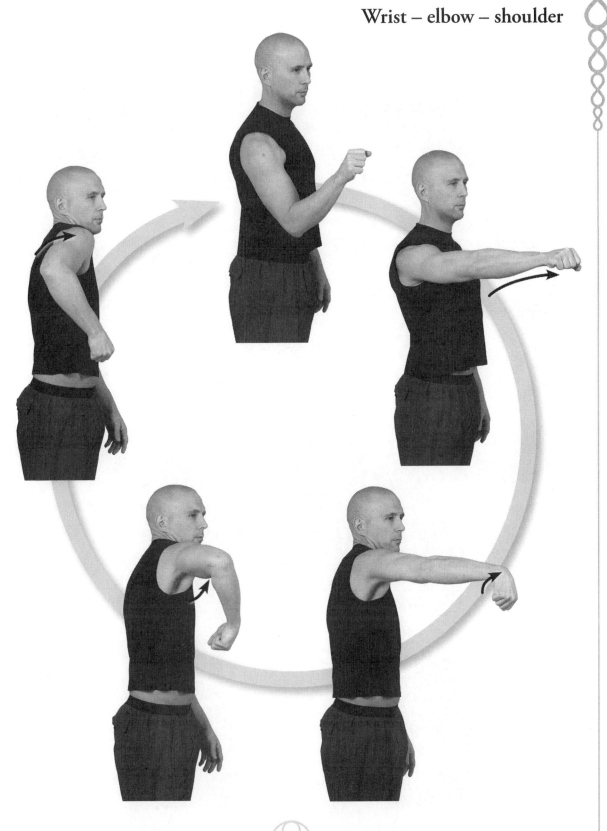

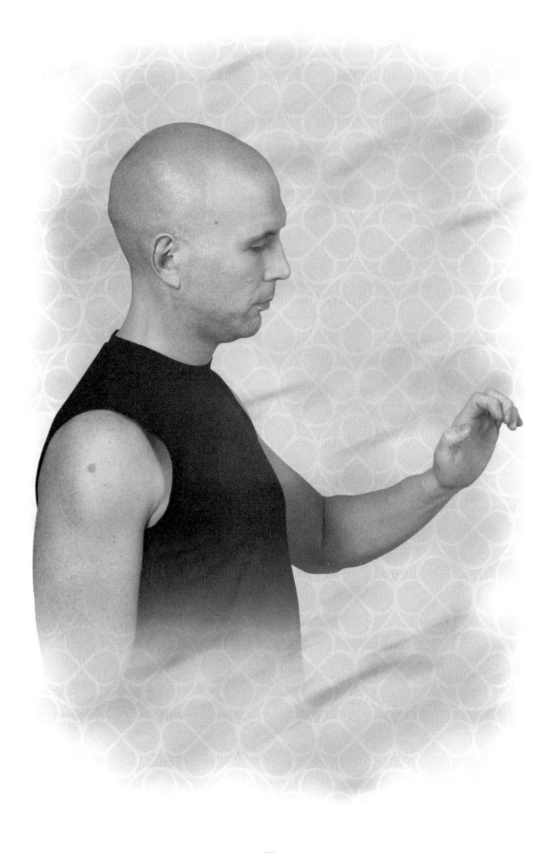

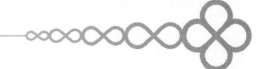

Wrists
Hands
Fingers

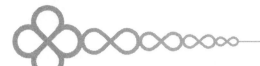

When not Free to Move from lack of prehabilitative movement due to stress, trauma, fear, overuse, underuse, or misuse, the following issues may result:

- Sprained and strained wrist
- Tendonitis
- Carpal tunnel syndrome
- Osteoarthritis
- Finger fracture

Common mental and emotional issues faced as a result of area not being Free to Move:

- Not being able to grasp or let go of the situation
- Feeling like you're not being given a hand
- Feeling like your hand has been slapped
- Difficulty handling experiences

Common organ referral affecting sensory-motor function of the area:

- There are no organs that refer pain directly to the wrist, hand, and fingers.
- While it is not technically organ referral, sometimes a neck problem (such as a herniated disc in the neck or a nerve entrapment syndrome) can cause wrist, hand, and finger pain.

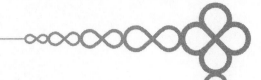

Wrist, hand, and finger mobility that will help you become Free to Move again:

17. **Ranges**
    a. Chopper
    b. Palm Strike
    c. Wrench Inside
    d. Wrench Outside

18. **Circles**
    a. Wrist: Top – right – bottom – left
    b. Wrist: Top – left – bottom – right
    c. Fingers: Each Clockwise and Counter-Clockwise

19. **Infinities**
    a. Left – top – right – left – bottom – right
    b. Right – top – left – right – bottom – left
    c. Top – right – bottom – top – left – bottom
    d. Bottom – right – top – bottom – left – top

20. **Diagonal infinities**
    a. Top – right – left – bottom – top
    b. Bottom – left – right – top – bottom
    c. Top – left – right – bottom – top
    d. Bottom – right – left – top – bottom

21. **Clovers**
    a. Top – right – left – top – bottom – left – right
       – bottom
    b. Bottom – right – left – bottom – top – left – right
       – top

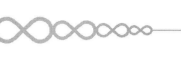

22. Waves
    a. Jellyfish: Wrist lift – first knuckle up – second knuckle up – third knuckle up/wrist down
    b. Gloving: Finger pad – second knuckle – first knuckle
    c. Okay – finger splay – ice cream cone

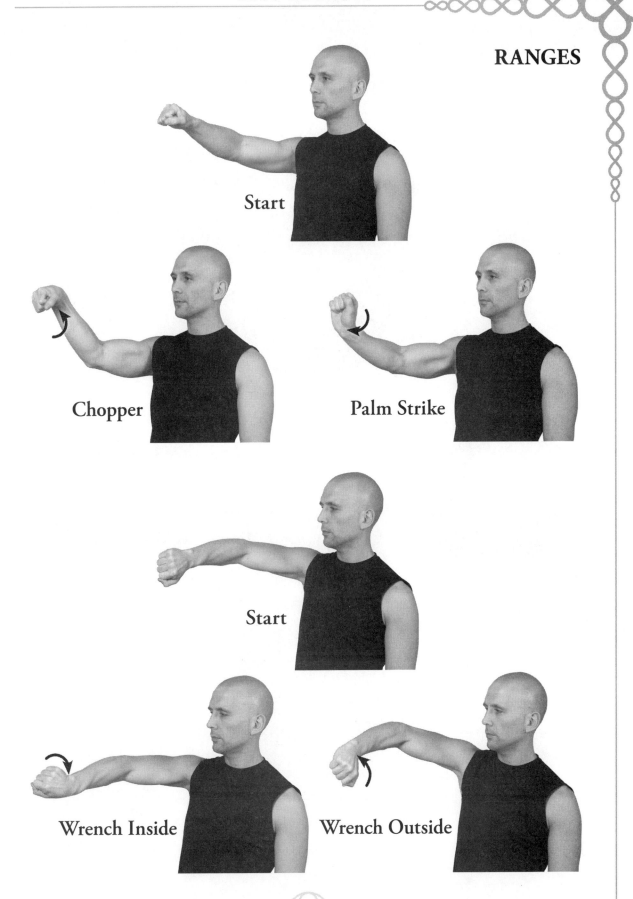

Start

Chopper

Palm Strike

Start

Wrench Inside

Wrench Outside

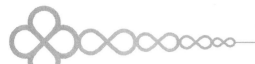

CIRCLES
Wrist: Top – right – bottom – left

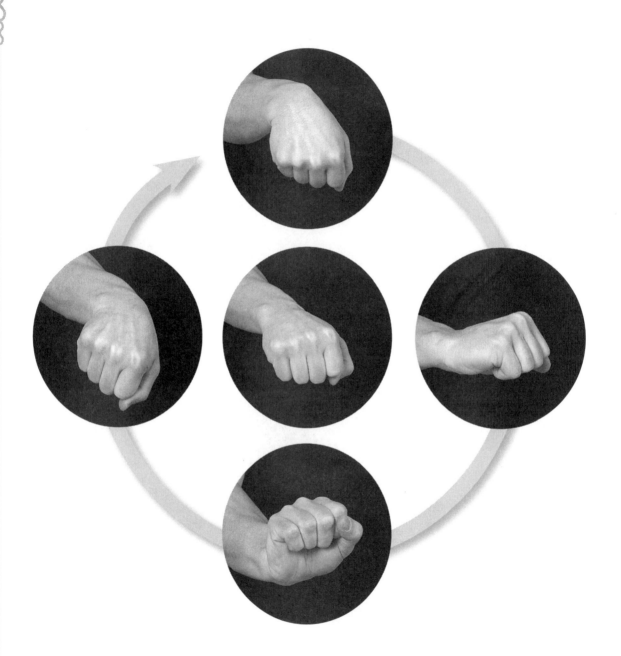

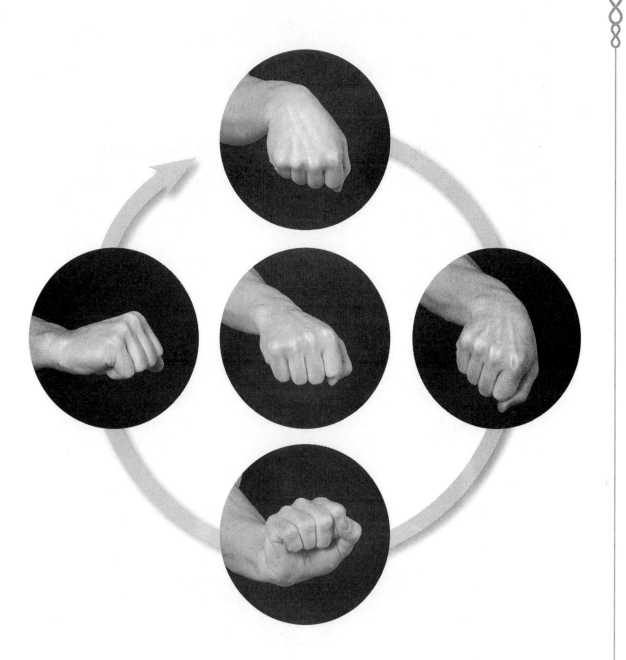

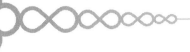

CIRCLES
Fingers: Each Clockwise and Counter-Clockwise

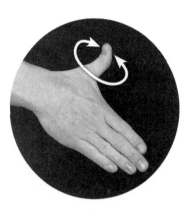

Thumb

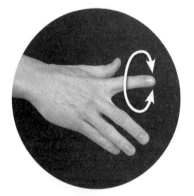

Index

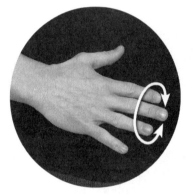

Middle

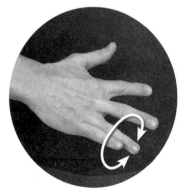

Ring

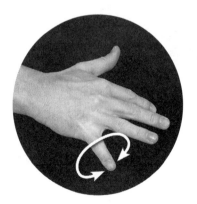

Pinky

INFINITIES
Left – top – right – left – bottom – right

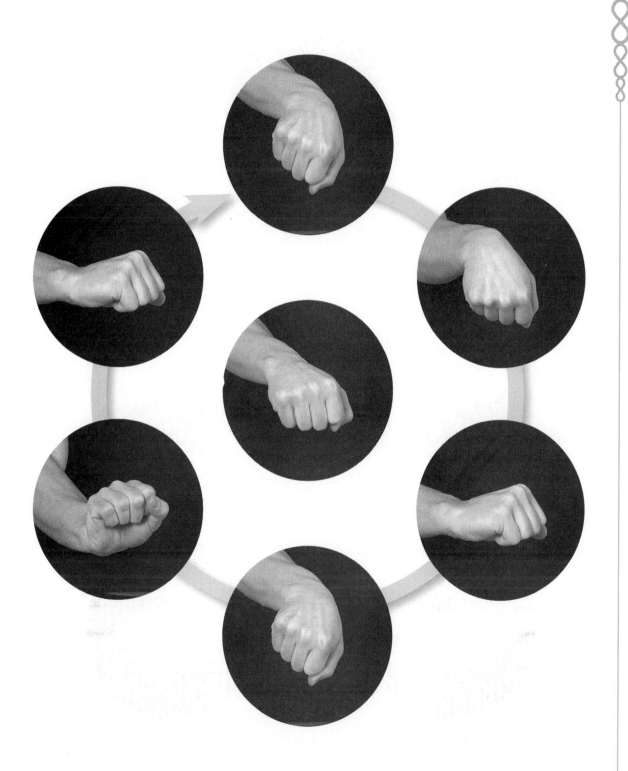

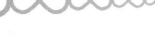

INFINITIES
Right – top – left – right – bottom – left

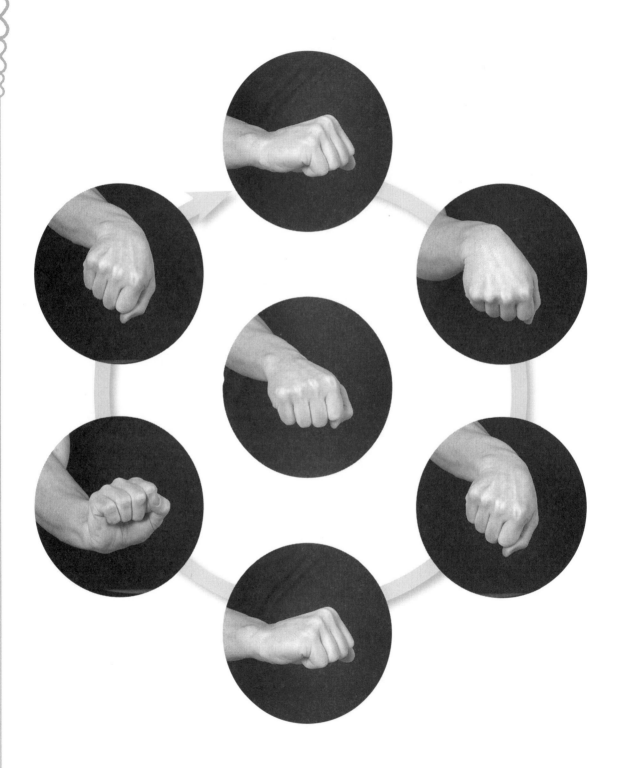

INFINITIES
Top – right – bottom – top – left – bottom

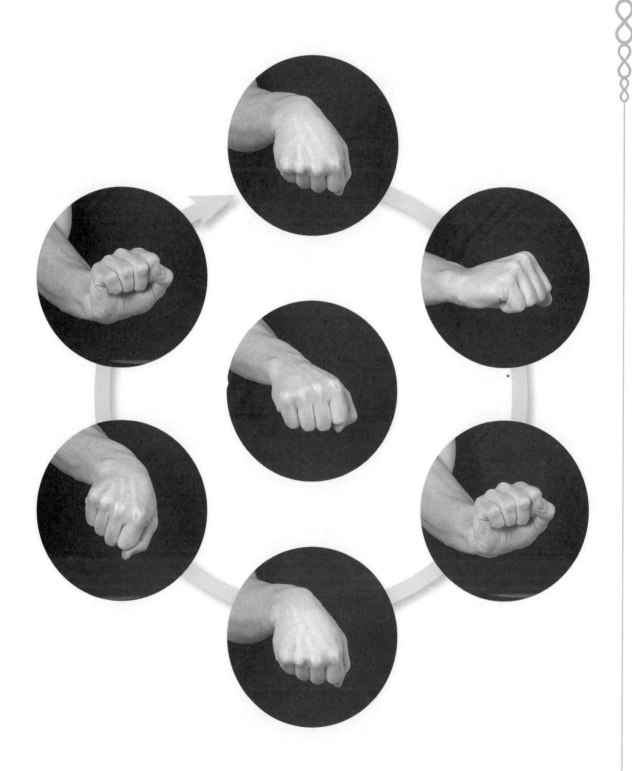

INFINITIES

Bottom – right – top – bottom – left – top

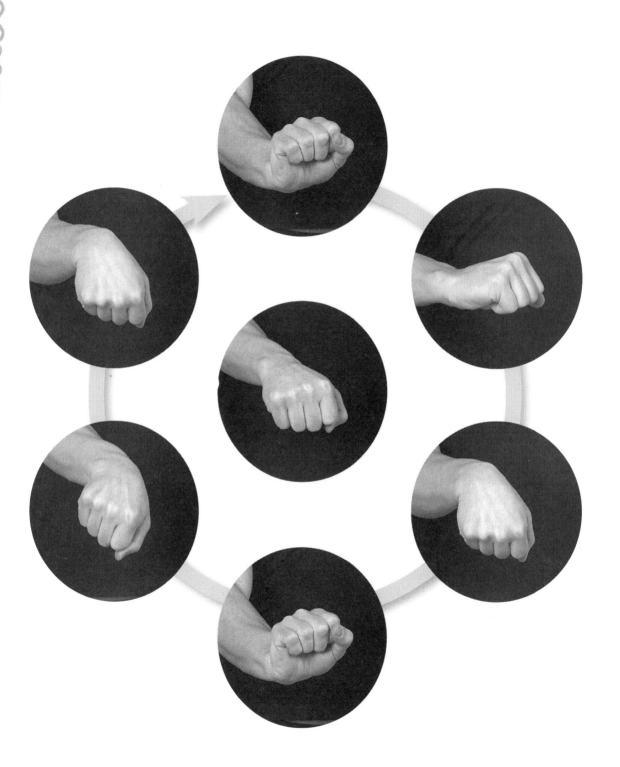

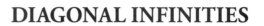

DIAGONAL INFINITIES
Top – right – bottom – top – left – bottom

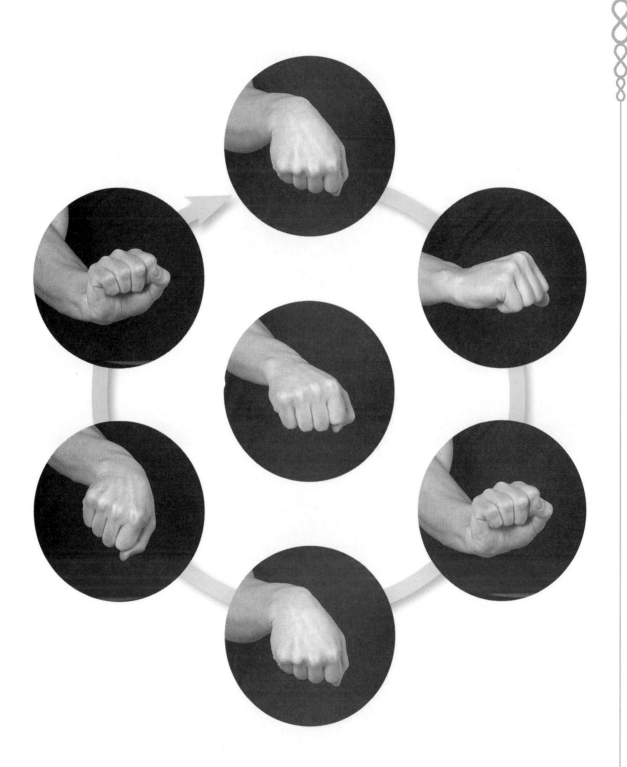

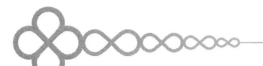

DIAGONAL INFINITIES
Bottom – left – right – top – bottom

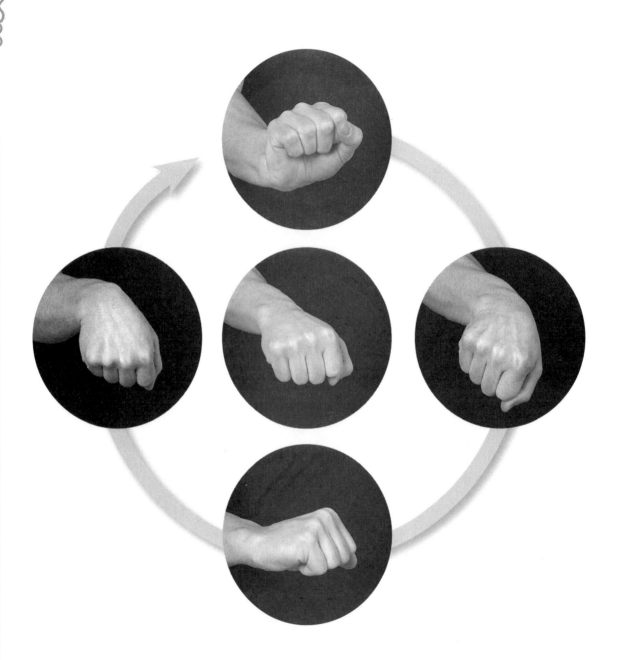

DIAGONAL INFINITIES
Top – left – right – bottom – top

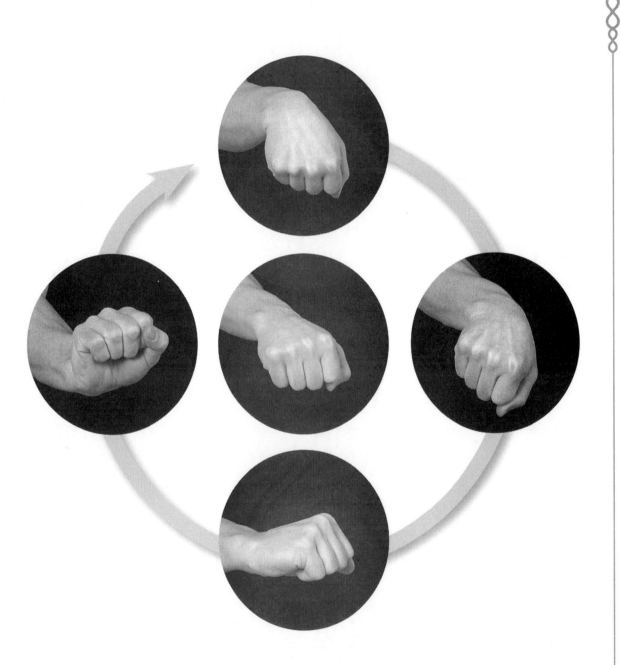

DIAGONAL INFINITIES
Bottom – right – left – top – bottom

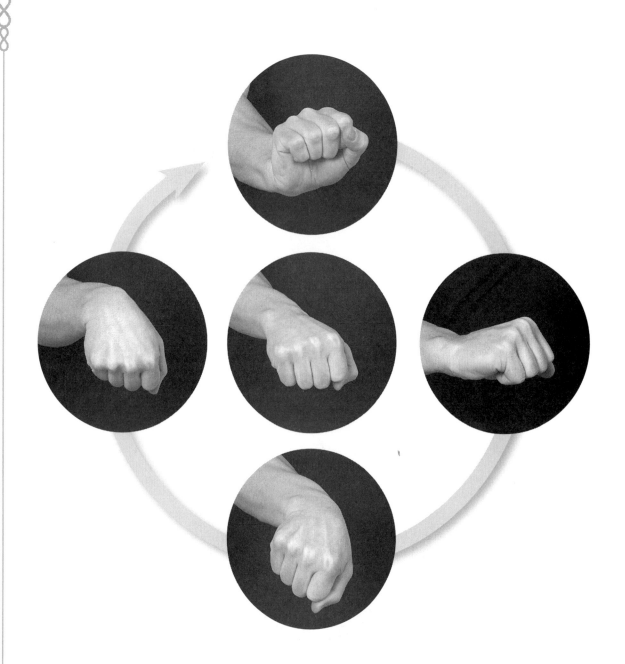

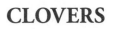

CLOVERS

Top – right – left – top – bottom – left – right – bottom

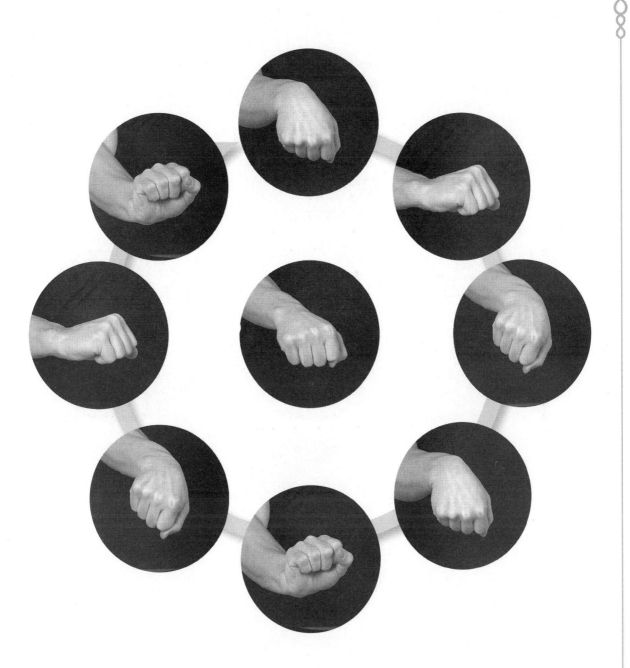

CLOVERS

Bottom – right – left – bottom – top – left – right – top

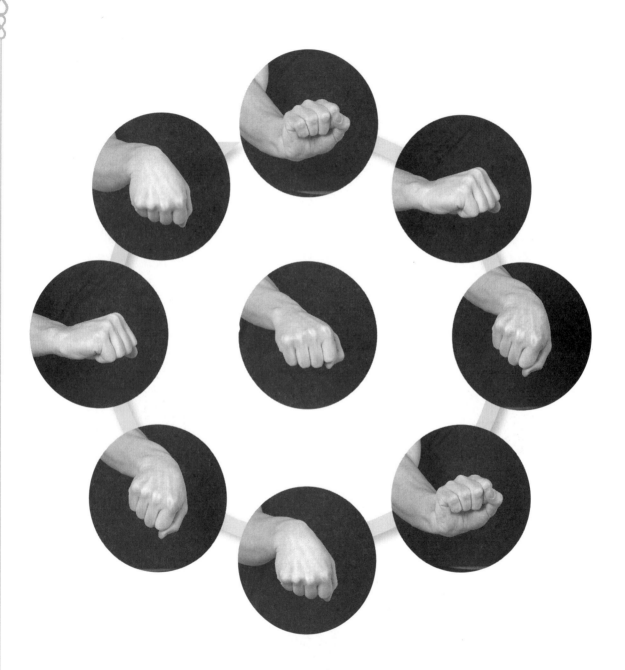

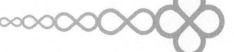

WAVES

Jellyfish: Wrist lift – first knuckle up – second knuckle up – third knuckle up/wrist down

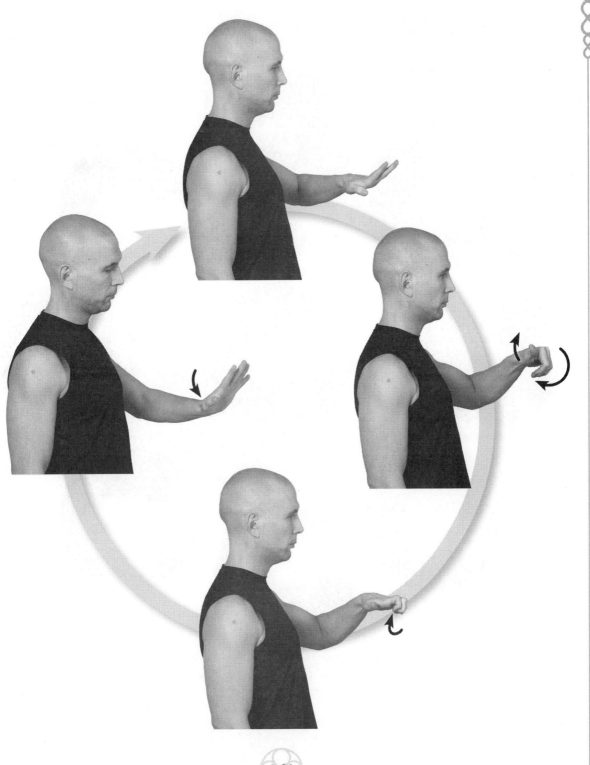

WAVES

Gloving: Finger pad – second knuckle – first knuckle

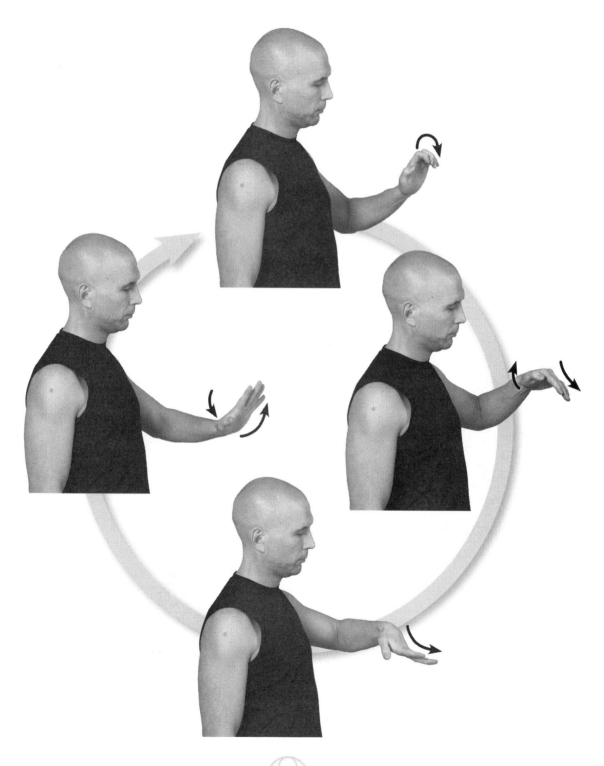

WAVES

Okay – finger splay – ice cream cone

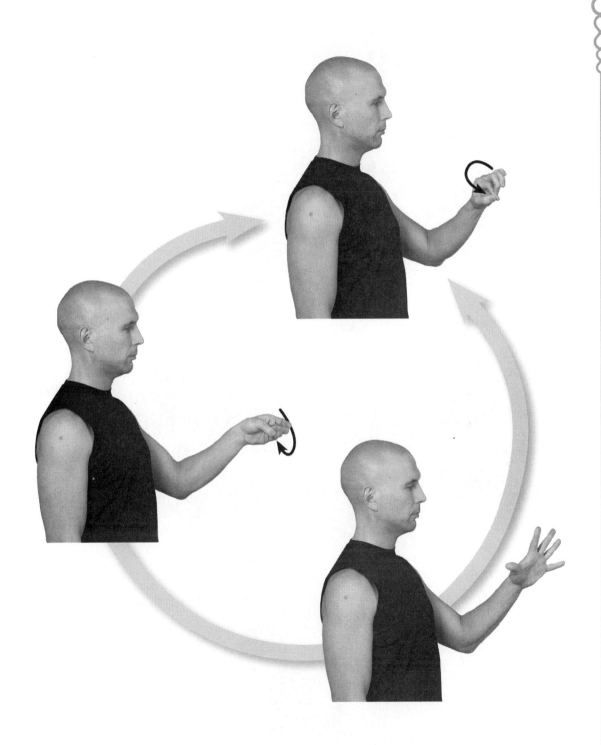

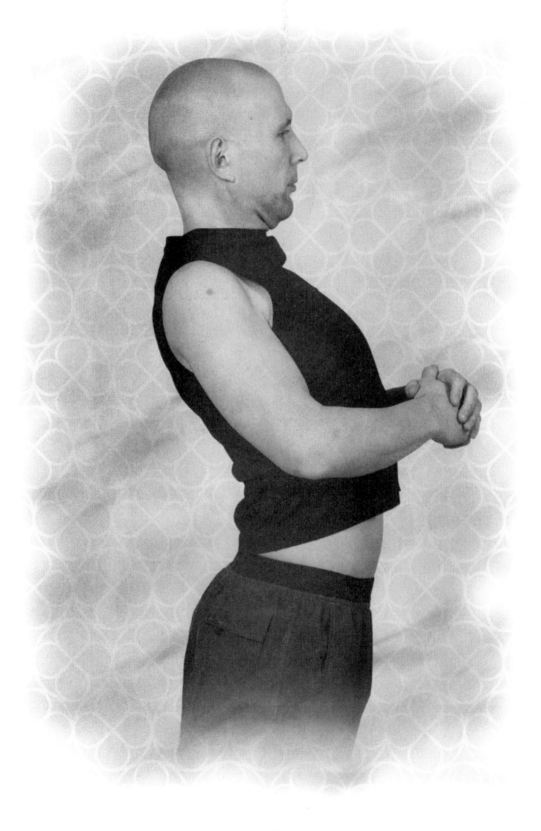

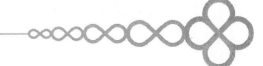

Mid Back

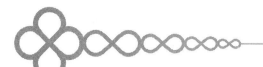

When not Free to Move from lack of prehabilitative movement due to stress, trauma, fear, overuse, underuse, or misuse, the following issues may result:

- Osteoarthritis
- Costochondritis
- Inflammation or injury involving the chest muscles
- Scoliosis
- Hyperkyphosis
- Hyperlordosis

Common mental and emotional issues faced as a result of area not being Free to Move:

- Feeling like you're vulnerable
- Feeling heartache
- Feeling stabbed in the back
- Feeling rage
- Mood swings between sorrow and anger

Common organ referral affecting sensory-motor function of the area:

- The gallbladder can refer pain to the right scapular (shoulder blade) region.
- The liver can refer pain or discomfort to the right side of the mid back.
- The stomach can refer pain or discomfort to the mid back and chest.
- The esophagus can refer pain or discomfort to the mid back and chest.
- The heart and large blood vessels can refer pain to the mid back and chest. (Heart attacks and aortic aneurysms are examples.)
- The lungs can refer pain to this area.

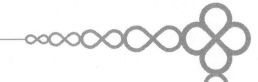

- The pancreas can also refer pain to the lower aspect of the mid back.
- The kidneys can refer pain to the lower aspect of the rib cage as well as to the lower back.
- The adrenal glands can refer pain to the lower mid back.

Thoracic mobility that will help you become Free to Move again:

23. **Ranges**
    a. Front
    b. Back
    c. Right
    d. Left
    e. Tai Chi Twist Left
    f. Tai Chi Twist Right

24. **Circles**
    a. Forward – right – backward – left
    b. Forward – left – backward – right

25. **Infinities**
    a. Left – forward – right – left – backward – right
    b. Right – forward – left – right – backward – left
    c. Forward – right – backward – forward – left – backward
    d. Backward – right – forward – backward – left – forward

26. **Diagonal infinities**
    a. Forward – right – left – backward – forward
    b. Backward – left – right – forward – backward
    c. Forward – left – right – backward – forward
    d. Backward – right – left – forward – backward

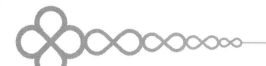
27. **Clovers**

    a. Forward – right – left – forward – backward – left – right – backward

    b. Backward – right – left – backward – forward – left – right – forward

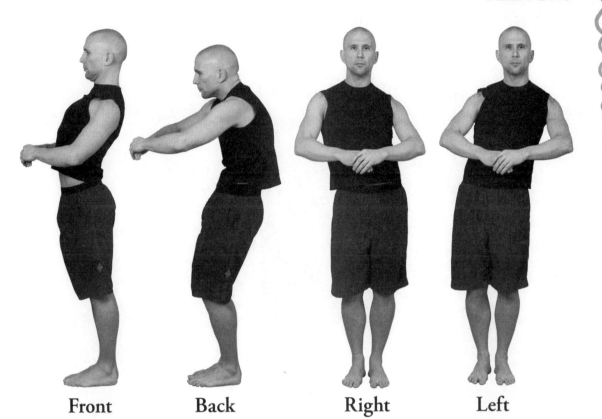

Front   Back   Right   Left

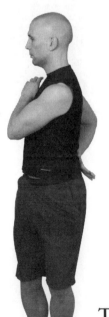
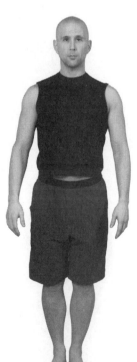
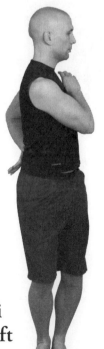

Tai Chi
Twist Right

Tai Chi
Twist Left

CIRCLES
Forward – right – backward – left

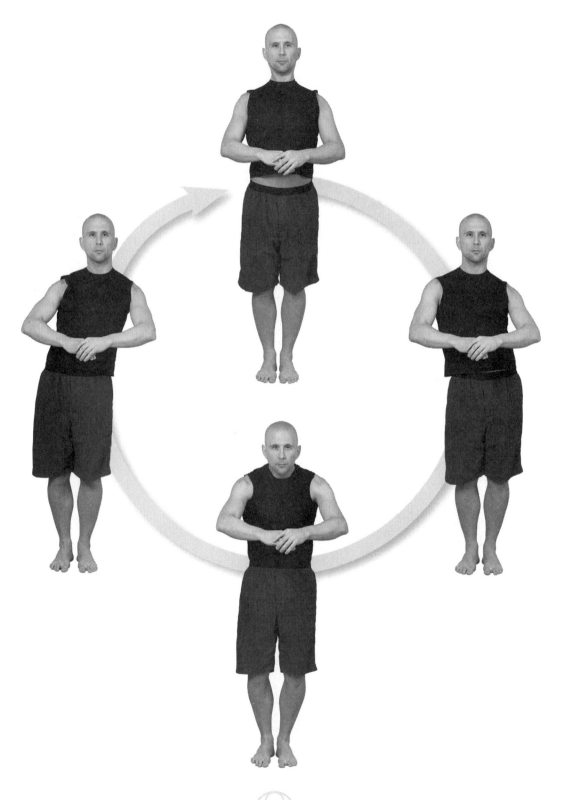

CIRCLES
Forward – left – backward – right

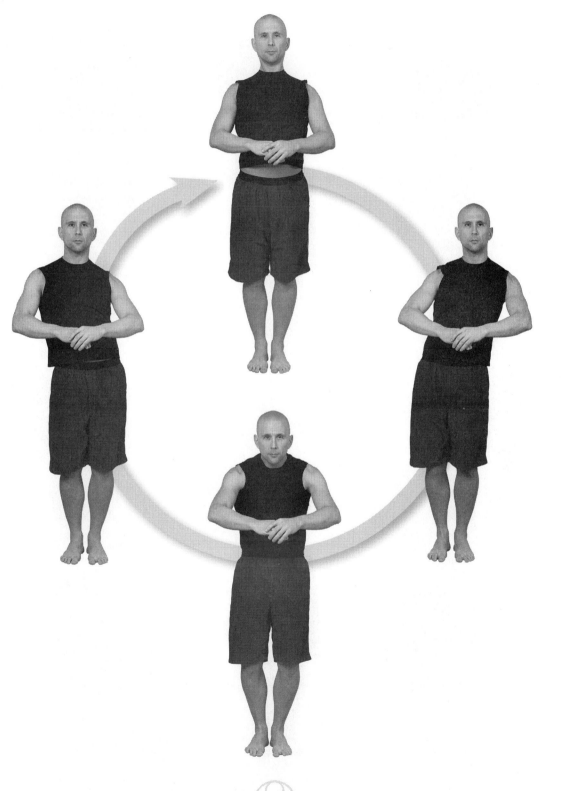

INFINITIES
Left – forward – right – left – backward – right

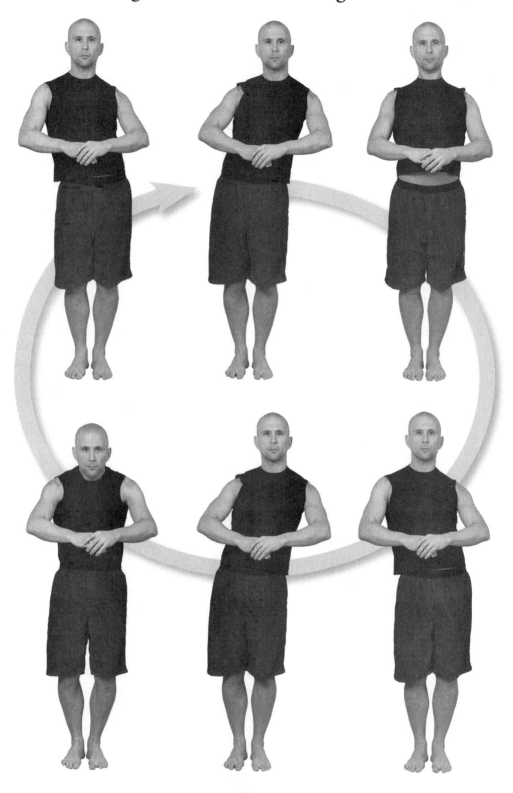

INFINITIES
Right – forward – left – right – backward – left

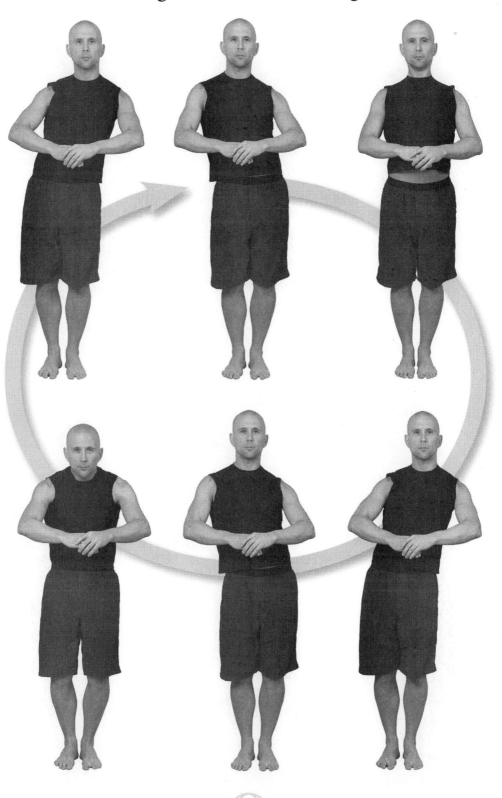

INFINITIES

Forward – right – backward – forward – left – backward

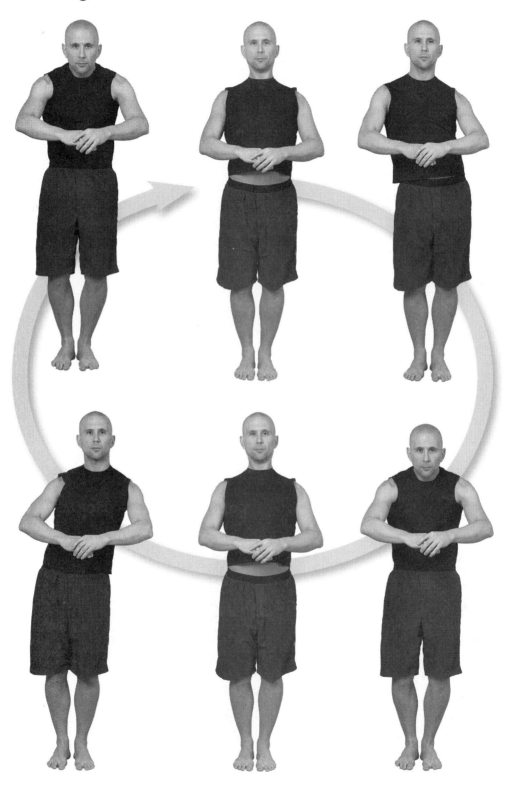

INFINITIES
Backward – right – forward – backward – left – forward

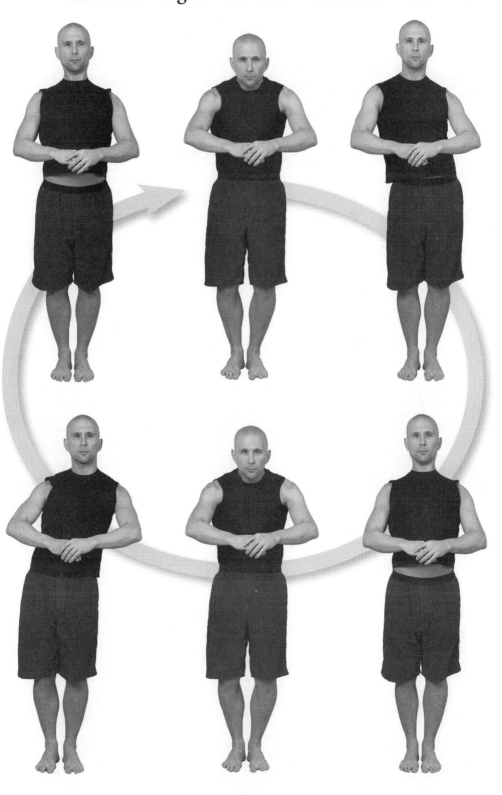

DIAGONAL INFINITIES

Forward – right – left – backward – forward

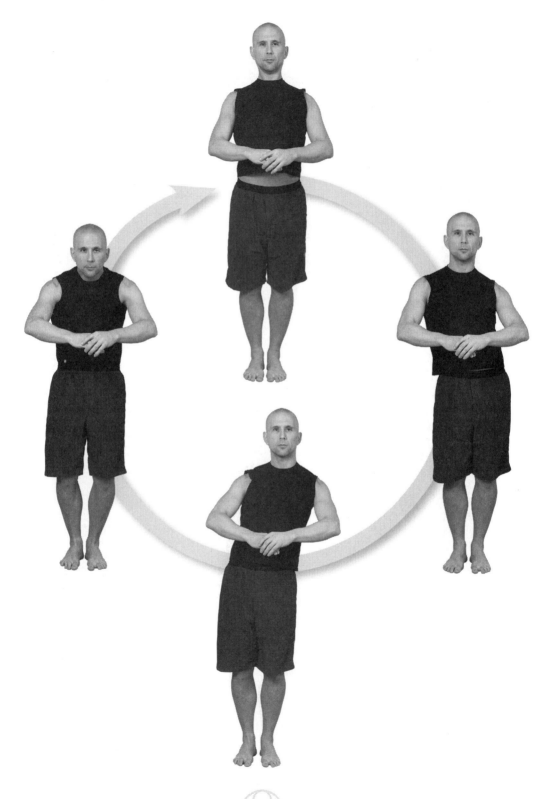

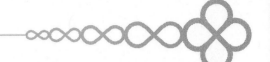

DIAGONAL INFINITIES
Backward – left – right – forward – backward

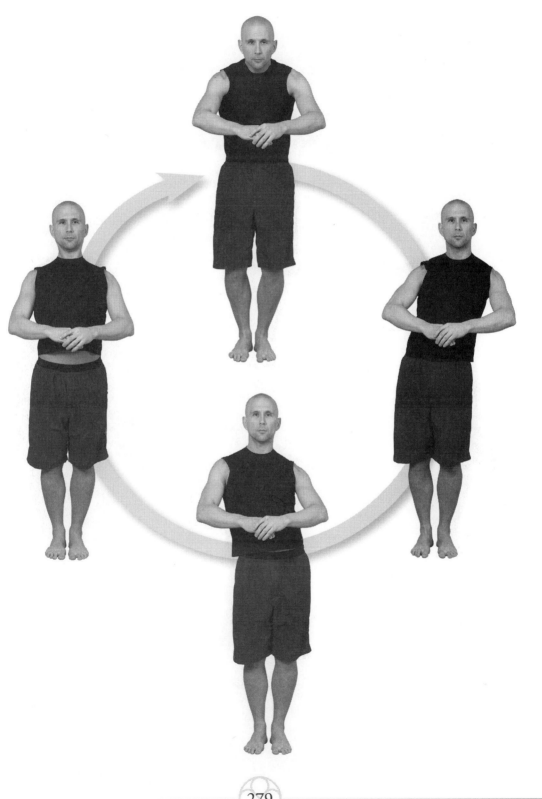

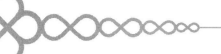

DIAGONAL INFINITIES

Forward – left – right – backward – forward

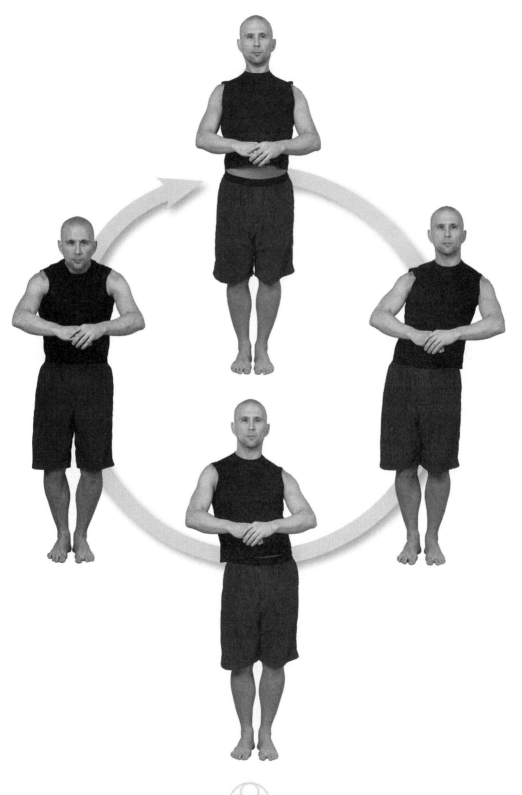

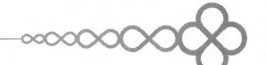

DIAGONAL INFINITIES
Backward – right – left – forward – backward

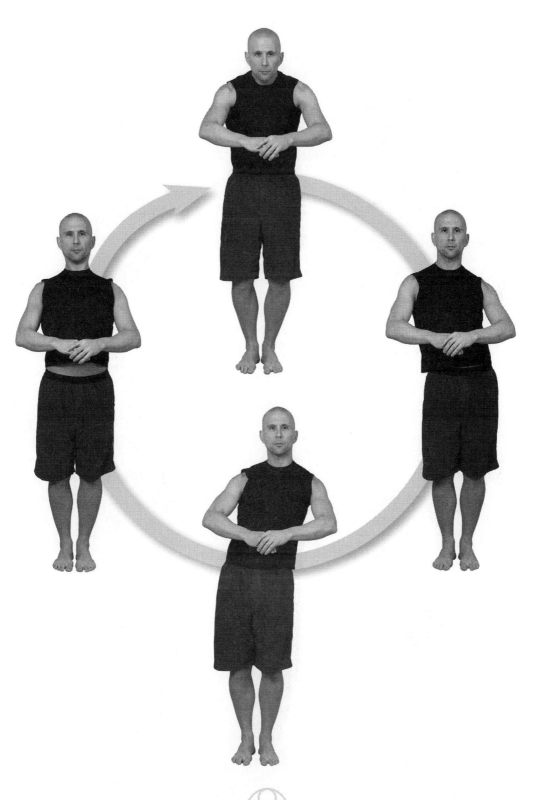

CLOVERS
Forward – right – left – forward – backward – left – right – backward

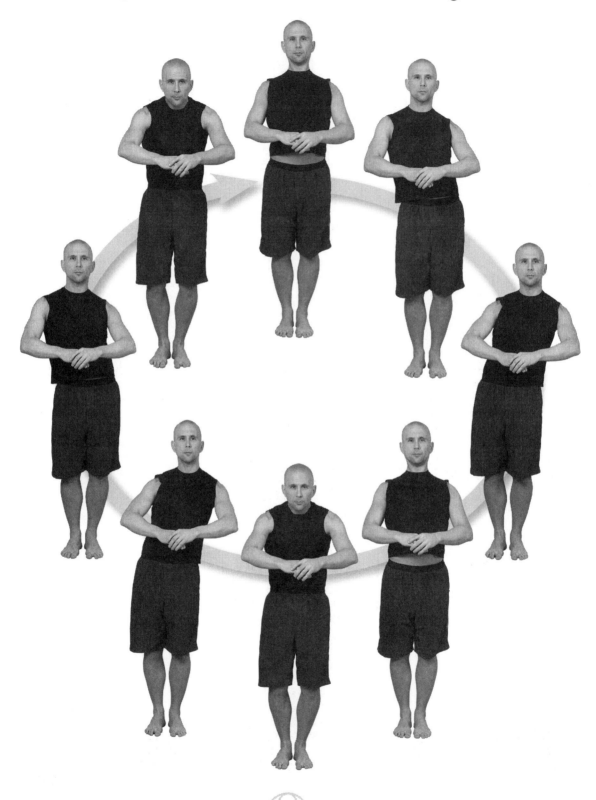

Backward – right – left – backward – forward – left – right – forward

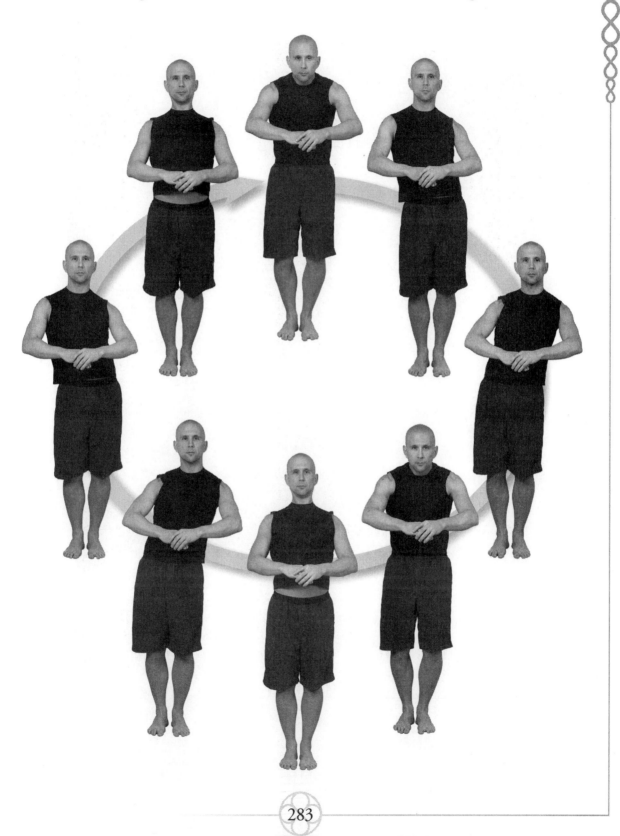

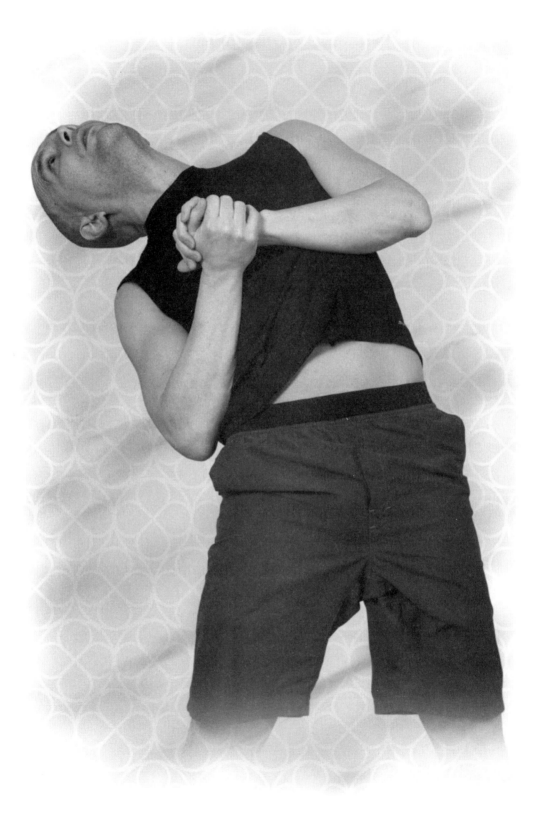

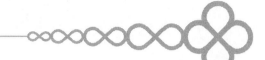

Lower Back

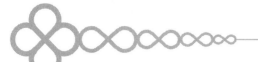

When not Free to Move from lack of prehabilitative movement due to stress, trauma, fear, overuse, underuse, or misuse, the following issues may result:

- Osteoarthritis
- Sciatica
- Lower back pain
- Scoliosis
- Hyperkyphosis
- Hyperlordosis

Common mental and emotional issues faced as a result of area not being Free to Move:

- Feeling unsupported
- Feeling insecure
- Lacking stability
- Lacking community development

Common organ referral affecting sensory-motor function of the area:

- The kidneys can refer pain to the lower aspect of the rib cage as well as to the lower back.
- The ureters (tubes running from your kidneys to your bladder) can refer pain to the lower back.
- The small and large colon can refer pain to the lower back.
- The appendix can refer pain to the lower back and pelvis.
- The ovaries, uterus, prostate, and bladder can also refer to the lower back and pelvis.
- Aortic aneurysms can cause pain in the lower back.

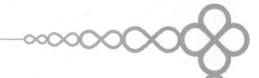

Lumbar mobility that will help you become Free to Move again:

28. **Ranges**
    a. Fold Forward
    b. Fold Backward
    c. Lean Right
    d. Lean Left

29. **Circles**
    a. Forward – right – backward – left
    b. Forward – left – backward – right

30. **Infinities**
    a. Left – forward – right – left – backward – right
    b. Right – forward – left – right – backward – left
    c. Forward – right – backward – forward – left – backward
    d. Backward – right – forward – backward – left – forward

31. **Diagonal infinities**
    a. Forward – right – left – backward – forward
    b. Backward – left – right – forward – backward
    c. Forward – left – right – backward – forward
    d. Backward – right – left – forward – backward

32. **Clovers**
    a. Forward – right – left – forward – backward – left – right – backward
    b. Backward – right – left – backward – forward – left – right – forward

33. **Waves**
    a. Down and Back: Shoulders – chest – hips lock – hips tilt
    b. Up and Forward: Hips tilt – hips lock – chest – shoulders

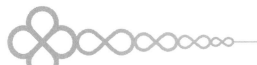

RANGES

Fold Forward

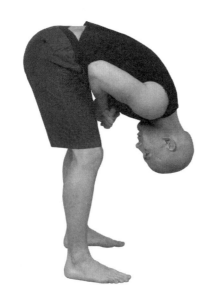

Fold Backward

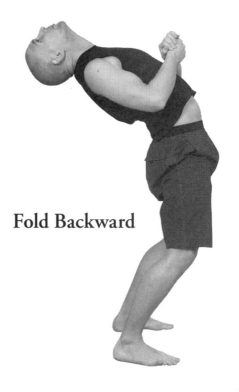

Lean Right

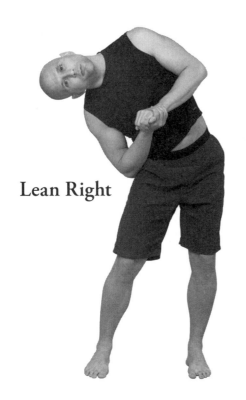

Lean Left

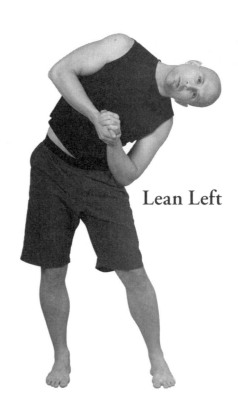

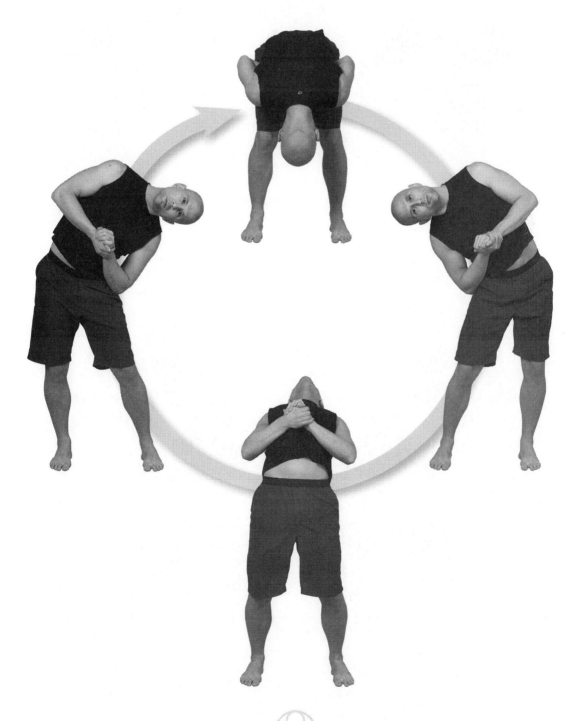

CIRCLES
Forward – left – backward – right

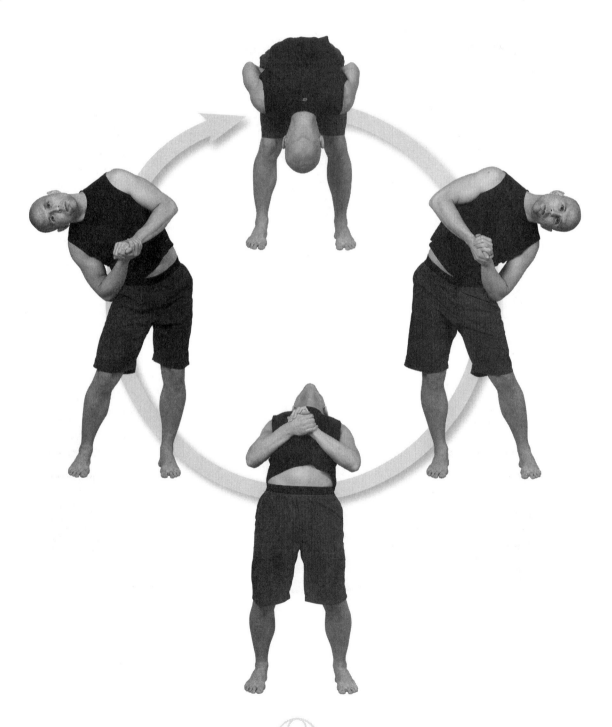

INFINITIES
Left – forward – right – left – backward – right

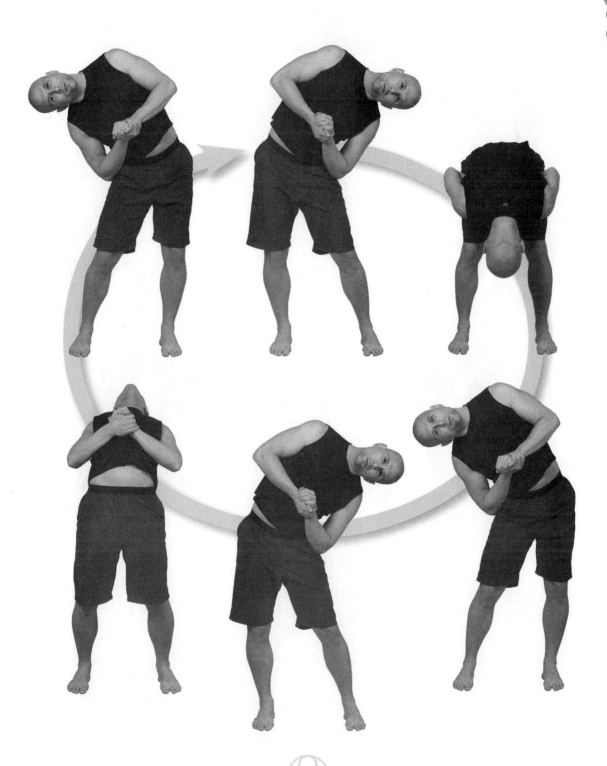

INFINITIES
Right – forward – left – right – backward – left

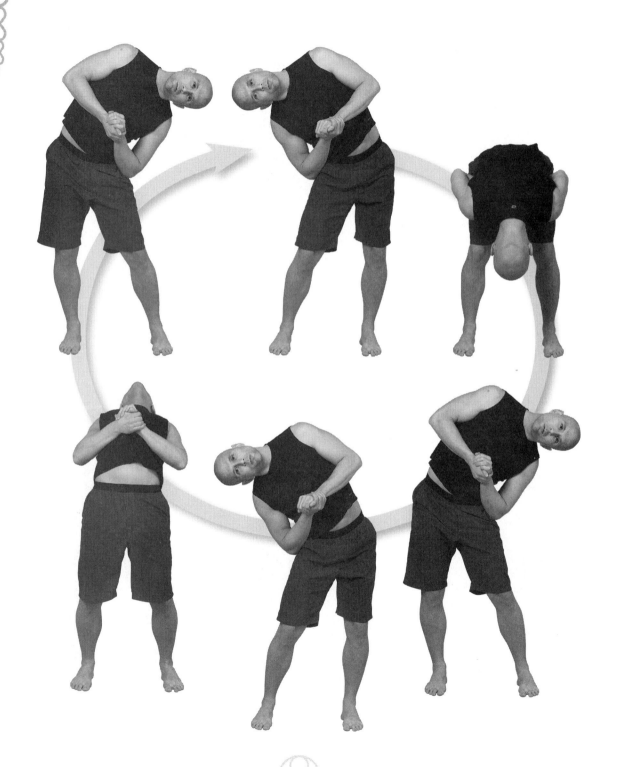

INFINITIES
Forward – right – backward – forward – left – backward

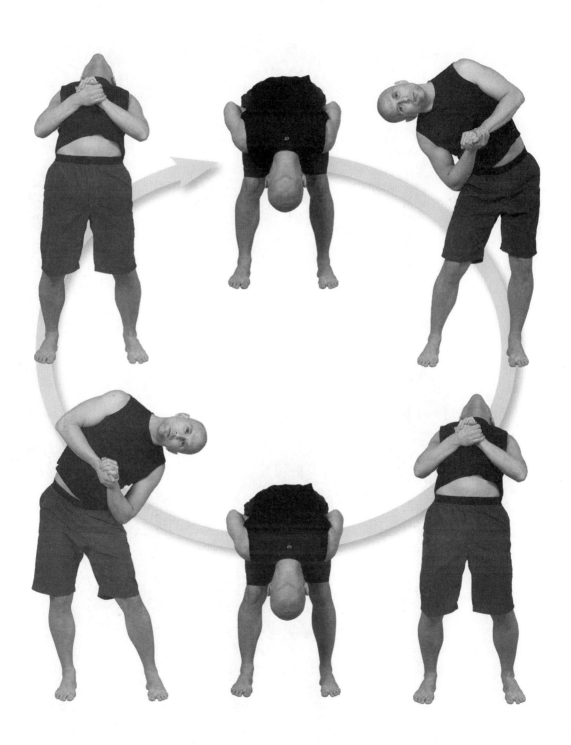

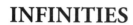

INFINITIES

Backward – right – forward – backward – left – forward

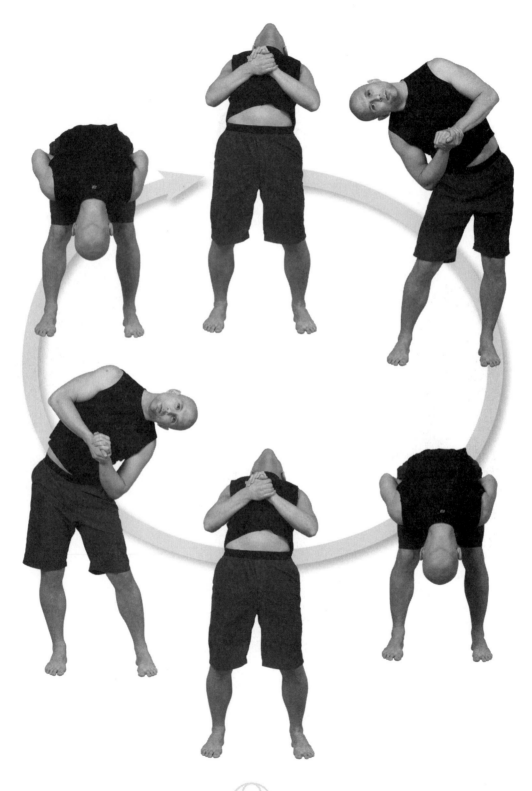

DIAGONAL INFINITIES
Forward – right – left – backward – forward

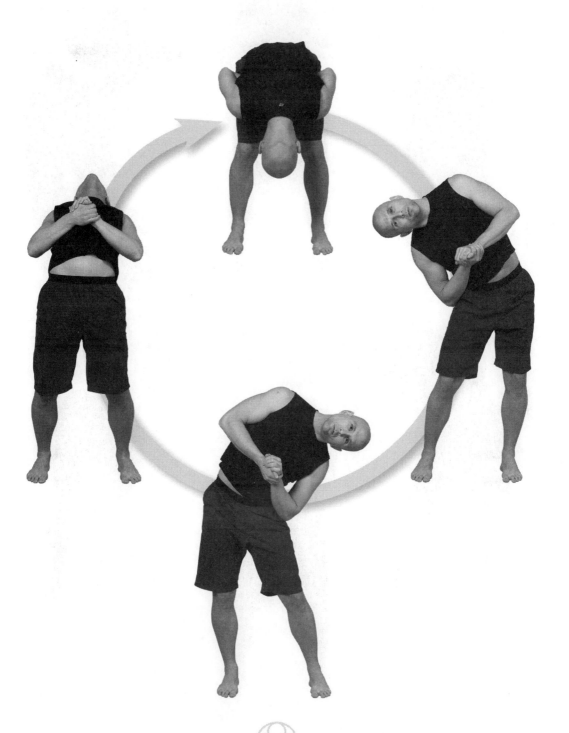

DIAGONAL INFINITIES

Backward – left – right – forward – backward

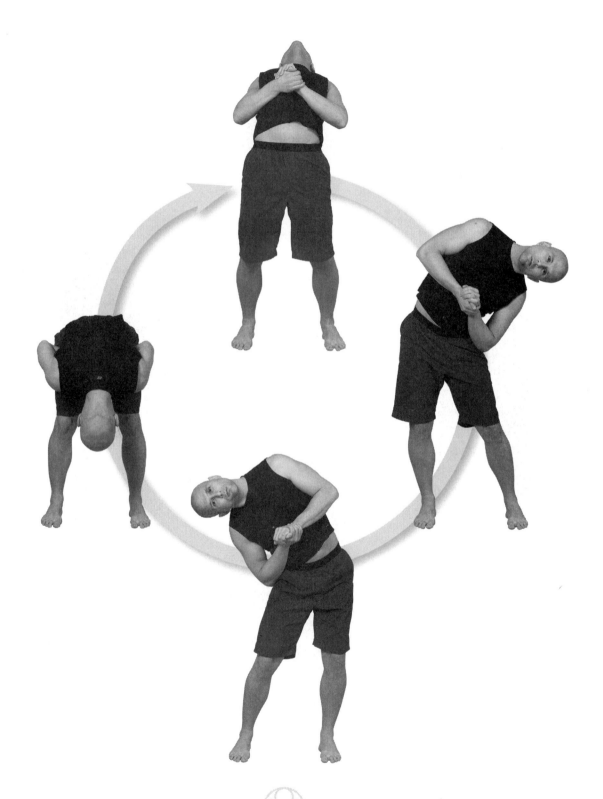

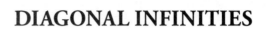

DIAGONAL INFINITIES
Forward – left – right – backward – forward

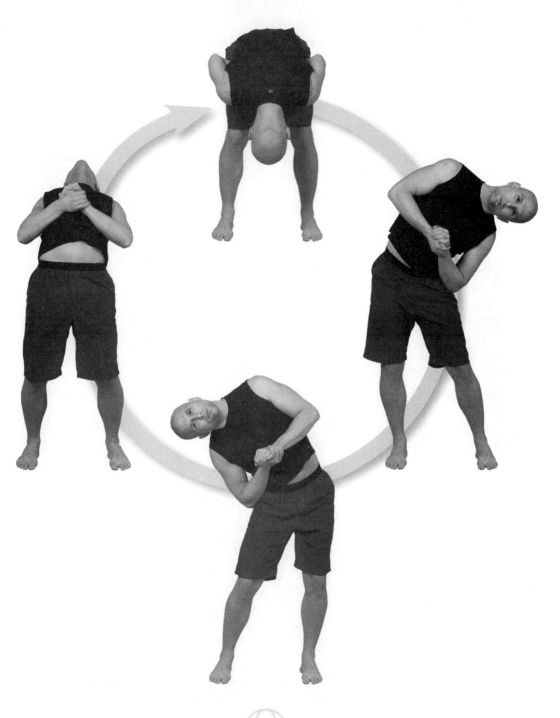

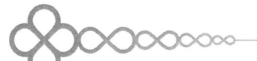

DIAGONAL INFINITIES

Backward – right – left – forward – backward

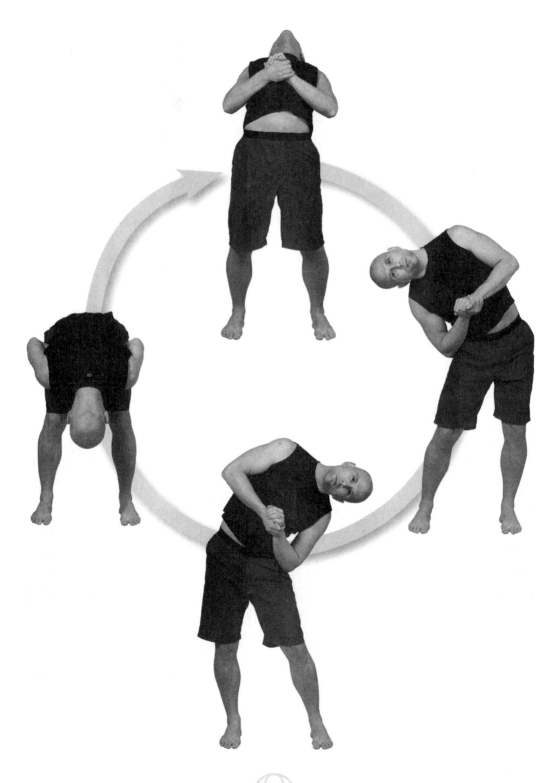

CLOVERS

Forward – right – left – forward – backward – left – right – backward

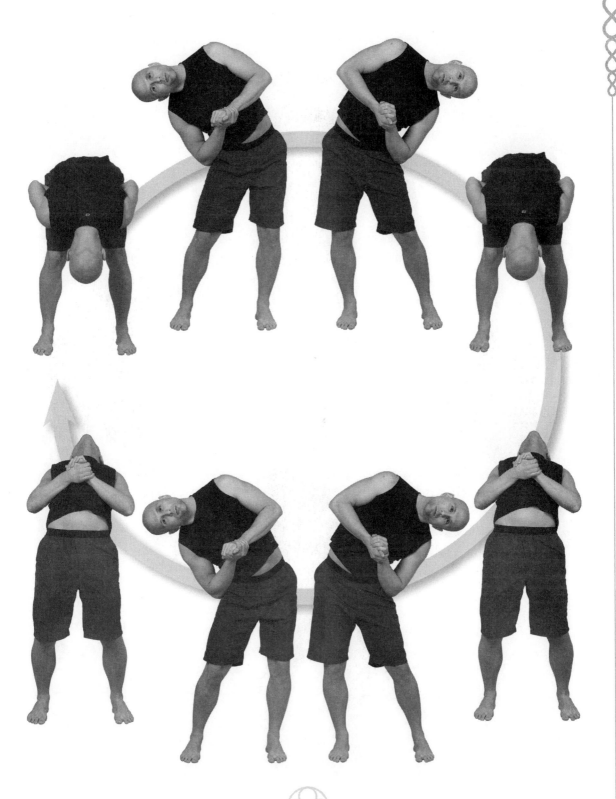

CLOVERS
Backward – right – left – backward – forward – left – right – forward

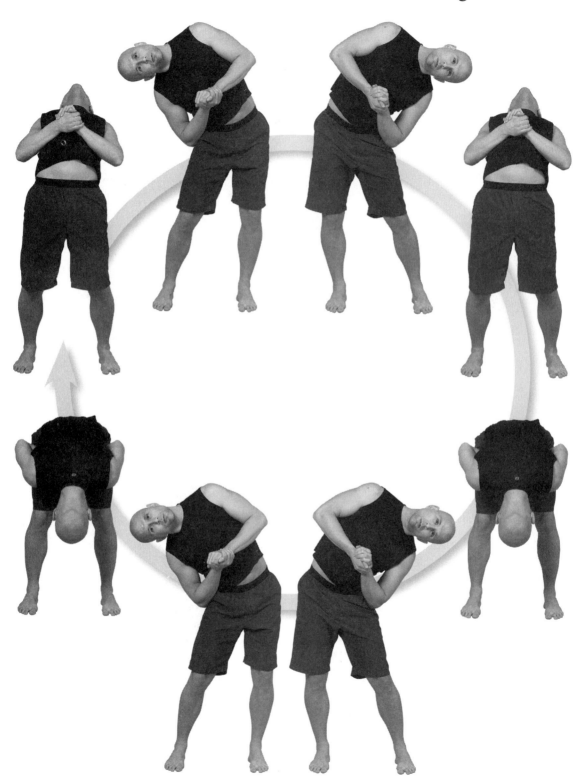

Down and Back: Shoulders – chest – hips lock – hips tilt

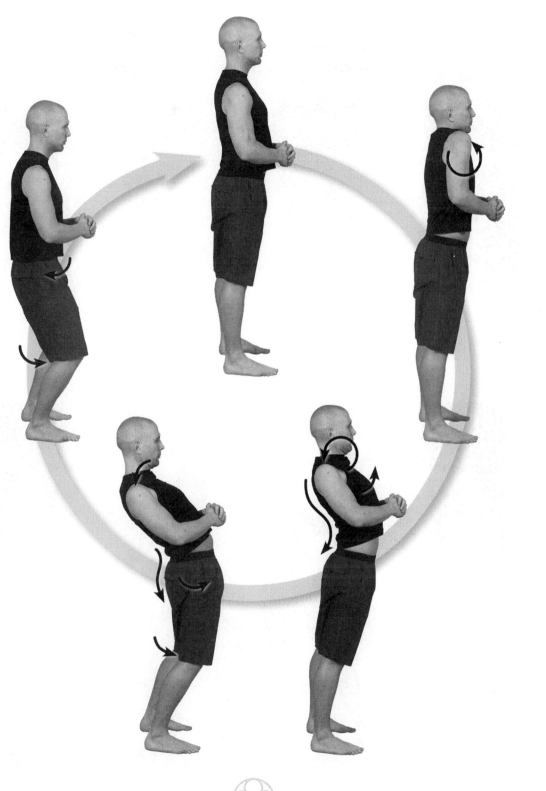

WAVES

Up and Forward: Hips tilt – hips lock – chest – shoulders

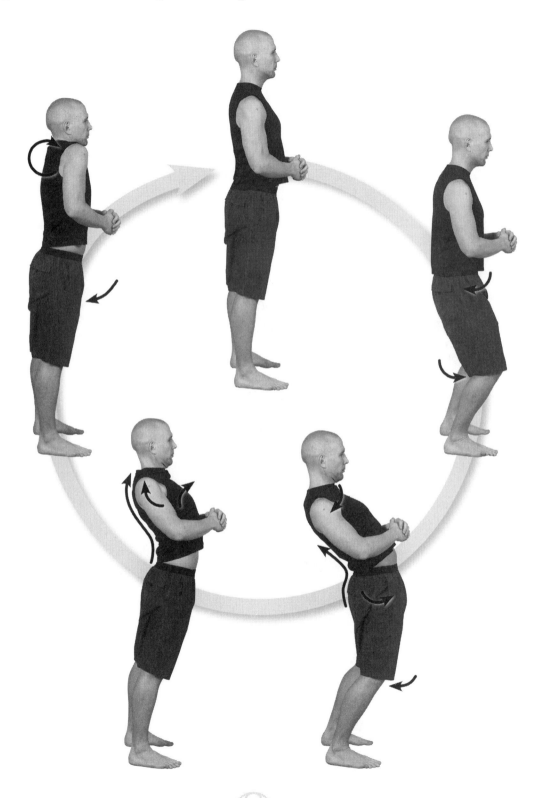

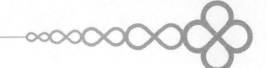

Pelvis & Hips

When not Free to Move from lack of prehabilitative movement due to stress, trauma, fear, overuse, underuse, or misuse, the following issues may result:

- Osteoarthritis
- Acute pelvic pain
- Chronic pelvic pain such as dysmenorrhea
- Hip pointer injury

Common mental and emotional issues faced as a result of area not being Free to Move:

- Feeling powerless
- Not wanting to let go of old anger or pain
- Feeling out of balance with yourself
- Blaming yourself for things out of your control

Common organ referral affecting sensory-motor function of the area:

- The rectum (an example would be hemorrhoids) can refer pain to this region.
- The appendix can refer pain to the lower back and pelvis.
- The ovaries, uterus, prostate, and bladder can also refer to the lower back and pelvis.
- The bladder refers pain to the pelvis, especially with infection or inflammation.
- The colon can also refer pain to the pelvis.
- The large blood vessels can refer pain to the pelvis. (Aneurysms are an example.)

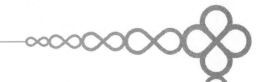

Pelvic mobility that will help you become Free to Move again:

34. **Ranges**
    a. Tilt Forward
    b. Tilt Backward
    c. Tilt Right
    d. Tilt Left

35. **Circles**
    a. Forward – right – backward – left
    b. Forward – left – backward – right

36. **Infinities**
    a. Left – forward – right – left – backward – right
    b. Right – forward – left – right – backward – left
    c. Forward – right – backward – forward – left – backward
    d. Backward – right – forward – backward – left – forward

37. **Diagonal infinities**
    a. Forward – right – left – backward – forward
    b. Backward – left – right – forward – backward
    c. Forward – left – right – backward – forward
    d. Backward – right – left – forward – backward

38. **Clovers**
    a. Forward – right – left – forward – backward – left – right – backward
    b. Backward – right – left – backward – forward – left – right – forward

39. **Waves**
    a. Mambo Backward and Forward

RANGES

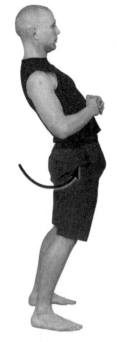
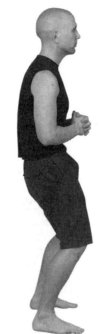
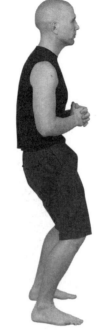

Tilt Forward   Tilt Backward

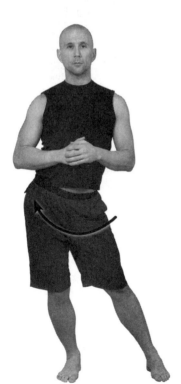
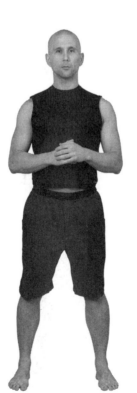
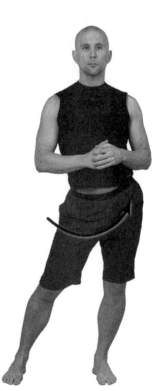

Tilt Right   Tilt Left

CIRCLES
Forward – right – backward – left

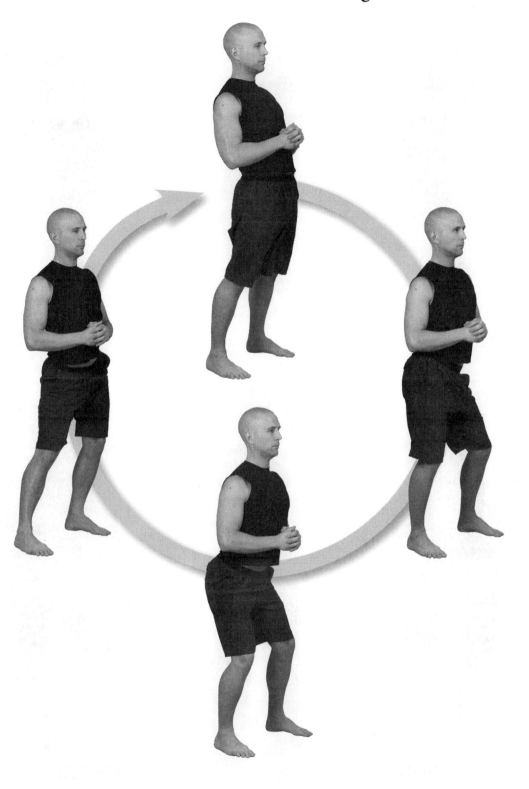

CIRCLES
Forward – left – backward – right

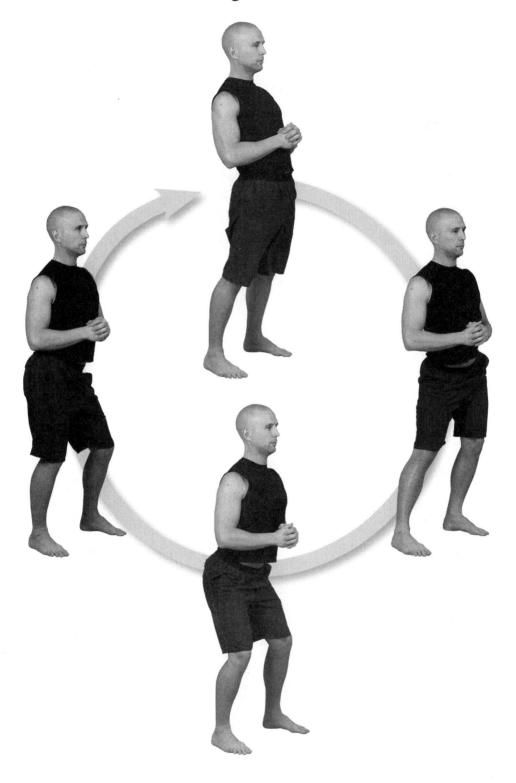

INFINITIES
Left – forward – right – left – backward – right

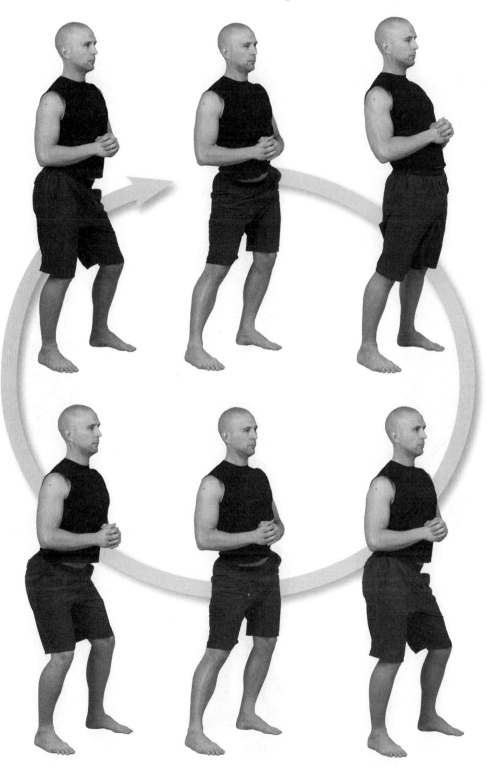

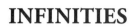

INFINITIES

Right – forward – left – right – backward – left

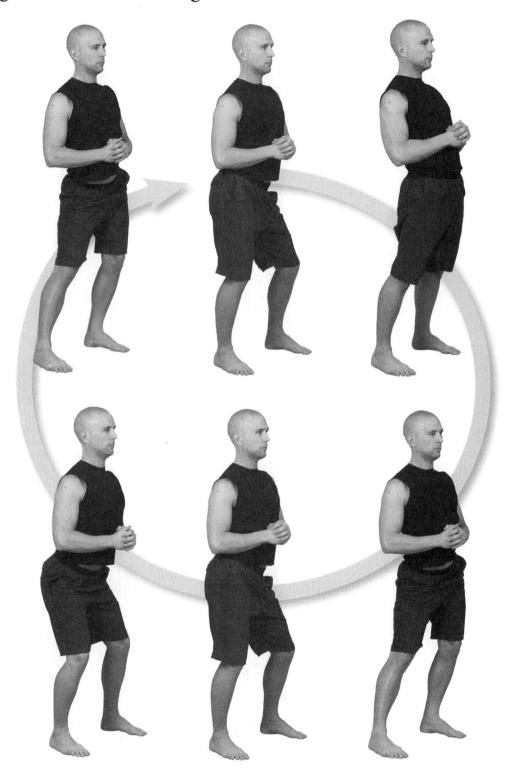

INFINITIES

Forward – right – backward – forward – left – backward

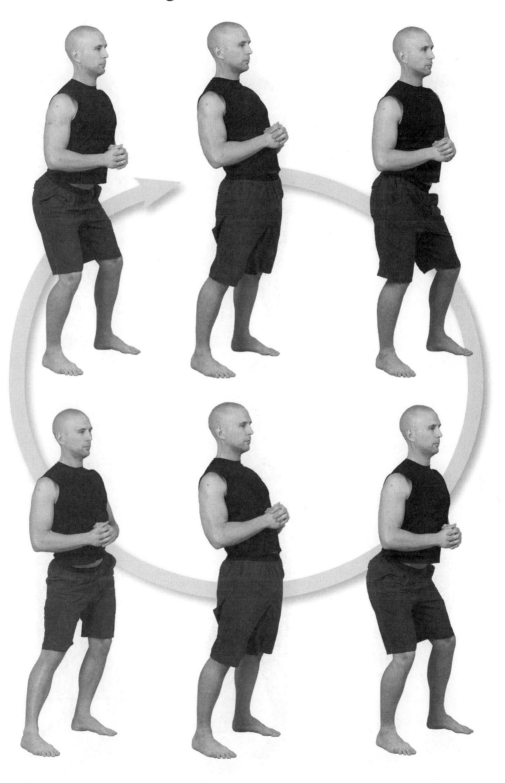

INFINITIES

Backward – right – forward – backward – left – forward

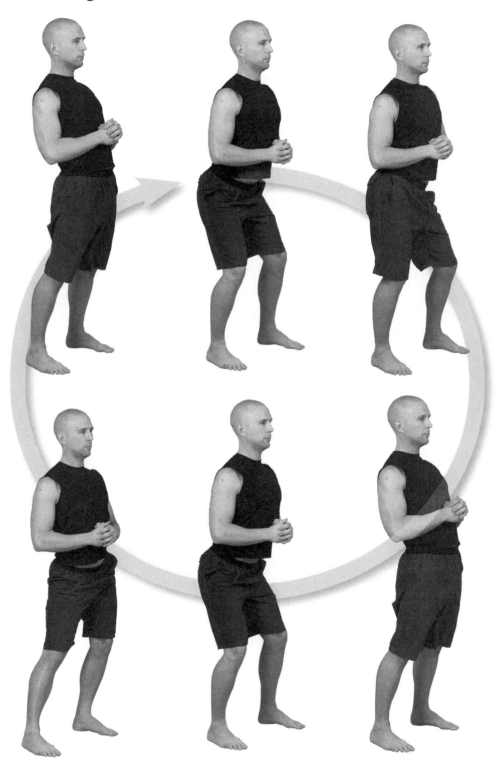

DIAGONAL INFINITIES

Forward – right – left – backward – forward

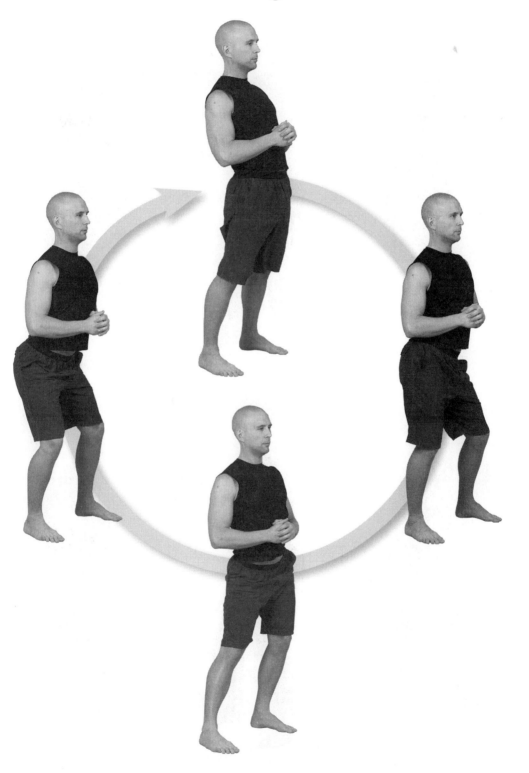

DIAGONAL INFINITIES

Backward – left – right – forward – backward

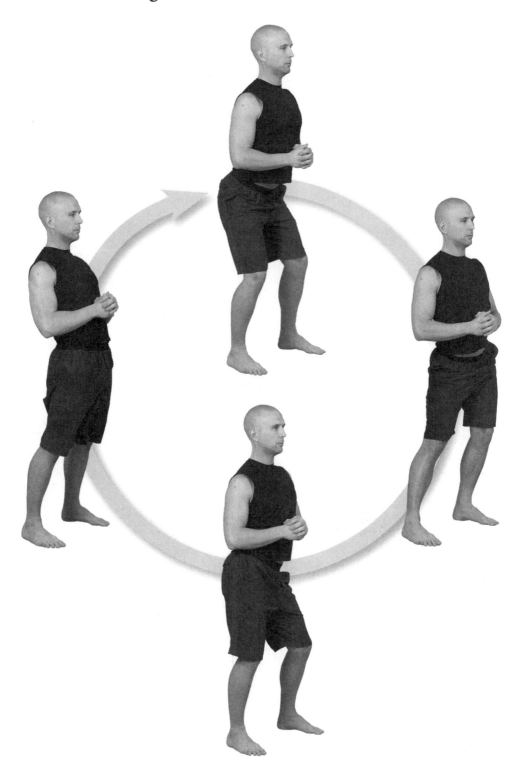

DIAGONAL INFINITIES
Forward – left – right – backward – forward

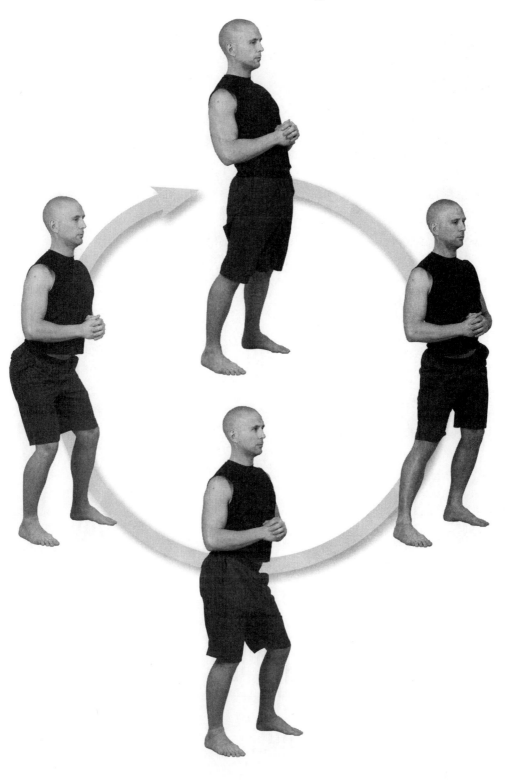

DIAGONAL INFINITIES
Backward – right – left – forward – backward

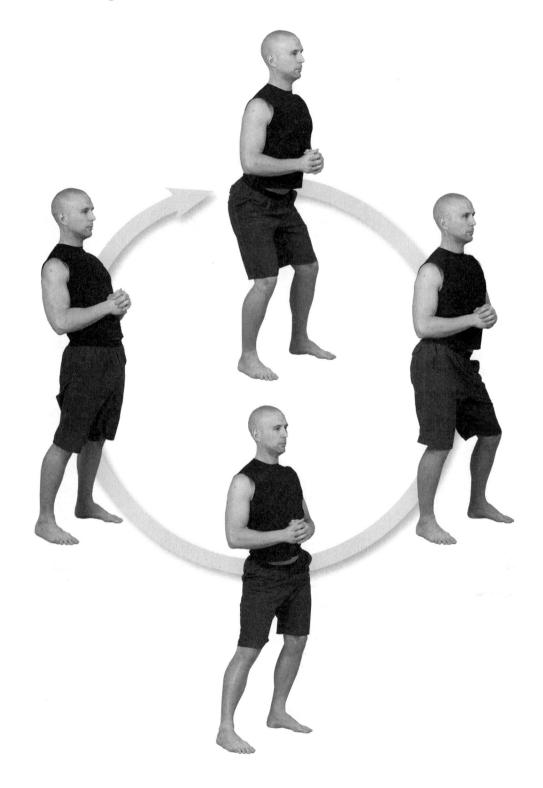

CLOVERS

Forward – right – left – forward – backward – left – right – backward

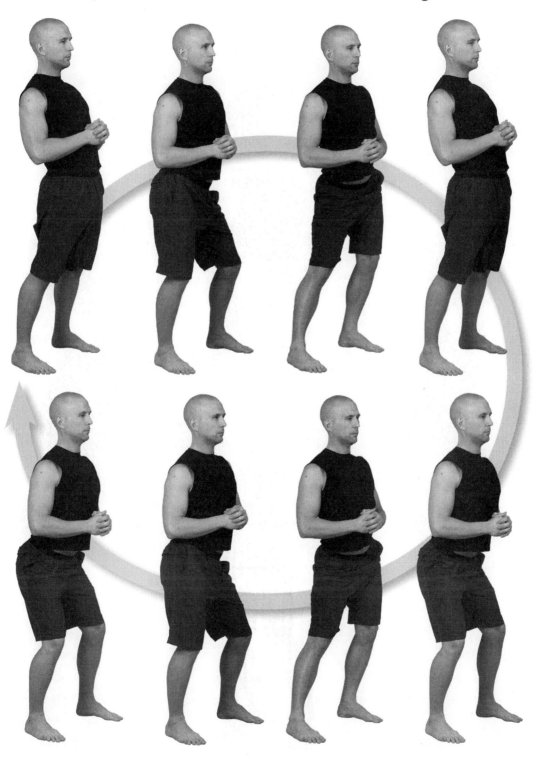

CLOVERS
Backward – right – left – backward – forward – left – right – forward

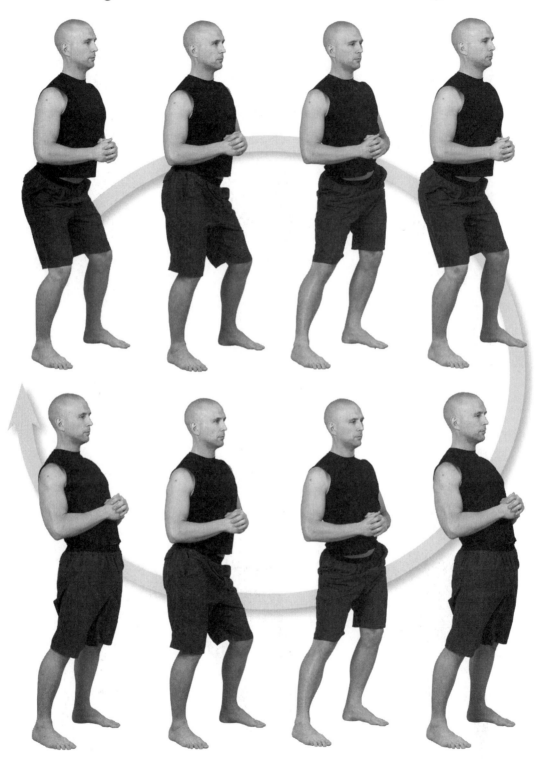

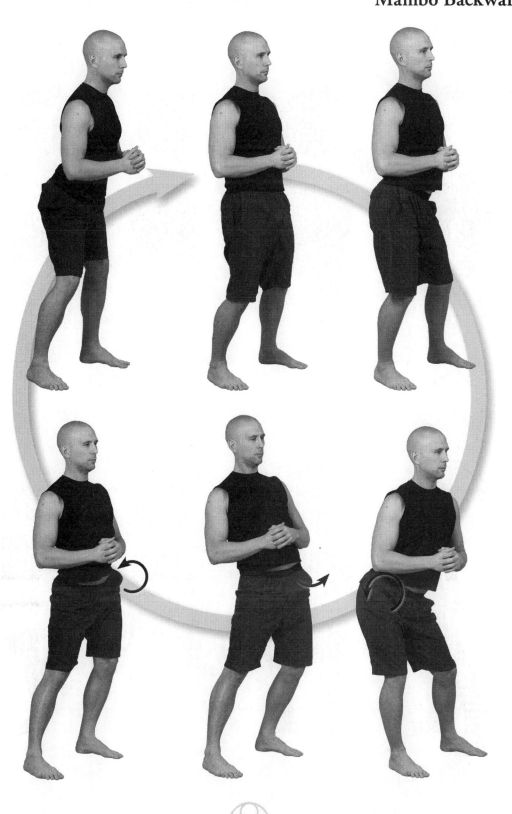

WAVES
Mambo Forward

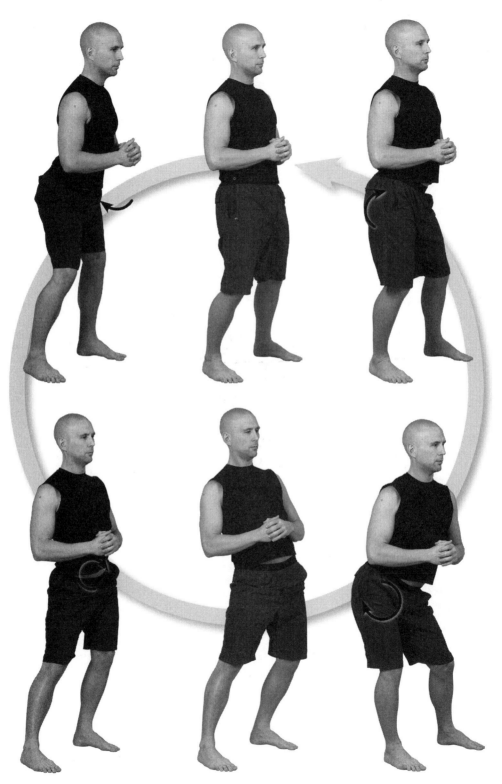

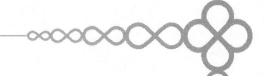

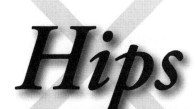

Hips

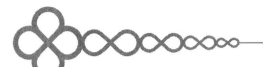

When not Free to Move from lack of prehabilitative movement due to stress, trauma, fear, overuse, underuse, or misuse, the following issues may result:

- Osteoarthritis
- Iliopsoas syndrome
- Piriformis syndrome

Common mental and emotional issues faced as a result of area not being Free to Move:

- Fear of moving forward with major decisions
- Fear that there is nothing to move forward to

Common organ referral affecting sensory-motor function of the area:

- Though it is not common, the ovaries, testicles, uterus, and prostate can refer pain to the hip region.
- While it is not technically organ referral, sometimes a lower back or pelvic problem (such as a herniated disc in the lower back or a nerve entrapment syndrome) can cause hip pain.

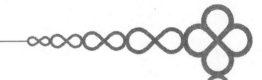

Hip mobility that will help you become Free to Move again:

40. **Ranges**
    a. Upward Dog
    b. Sleeping Warrior
    c. Spinal Twist
    d. Straddle Bent-Knee

41. **Circles**
    a. Front Clockwise and Counter-Clockwise
    b. Back Clockwise and Counter-Clockwise
    c. Inside Clockwise and Counter-Clockwise
    d. Outside Clockwise and Counter-Clockwise

42. **Infinities**
    a. Front – Back
    b. Back – Front
    c. Inside – Outside
    d. Outside – Inside

RANGES

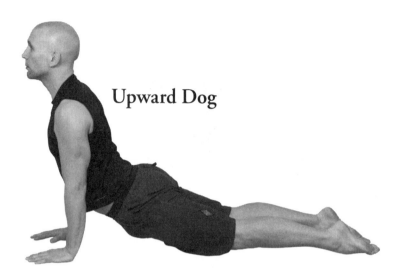

Upward Dog

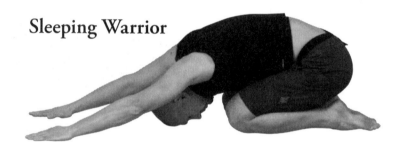

Sleeping Warrior

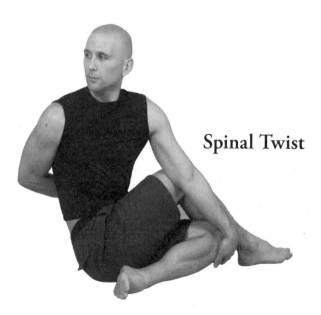

Spinal Twist

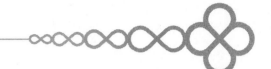

Straddle Bent-Knee Forward

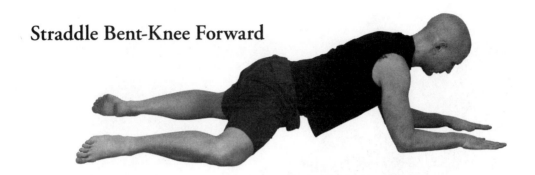

Straddle Bent-Knee Middle

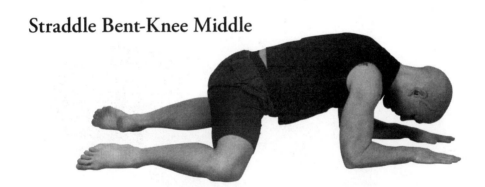

Straddle Bent-Knee Back

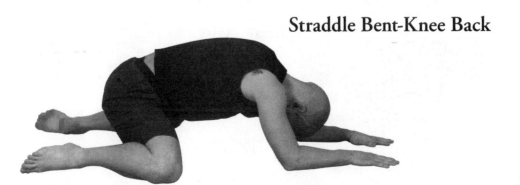

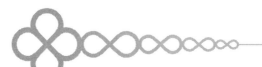

CIRCLES
Front Clockwise

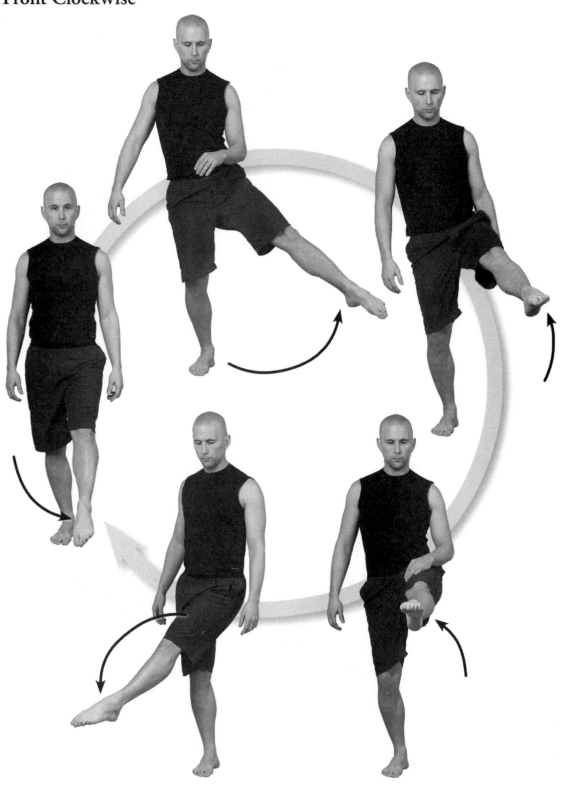

CIRCLES
Front Counter-Clockwise

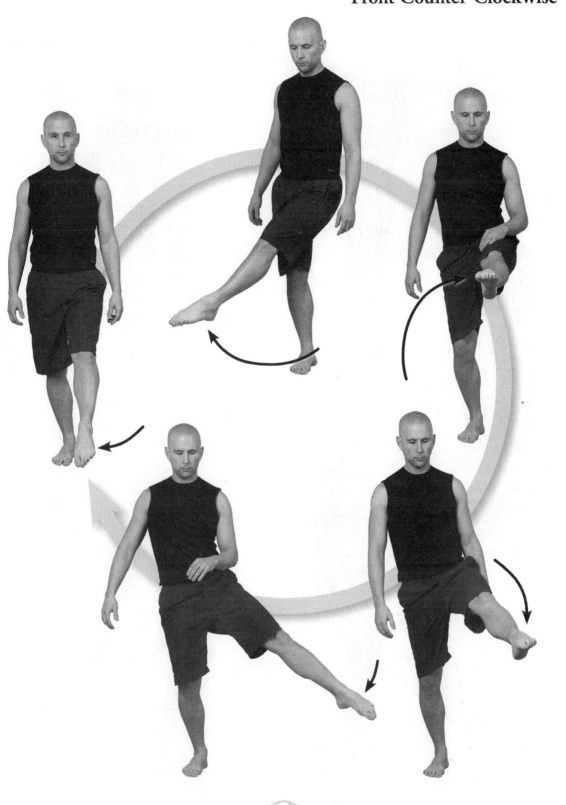

CIRCLES
Back Clockwise

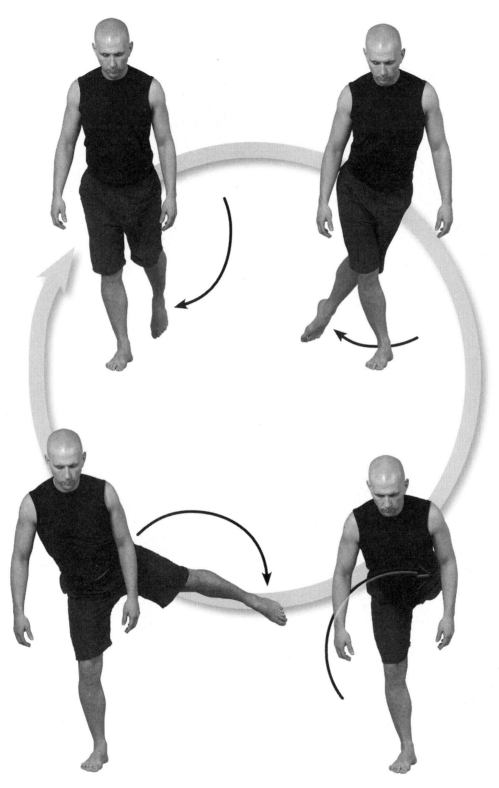

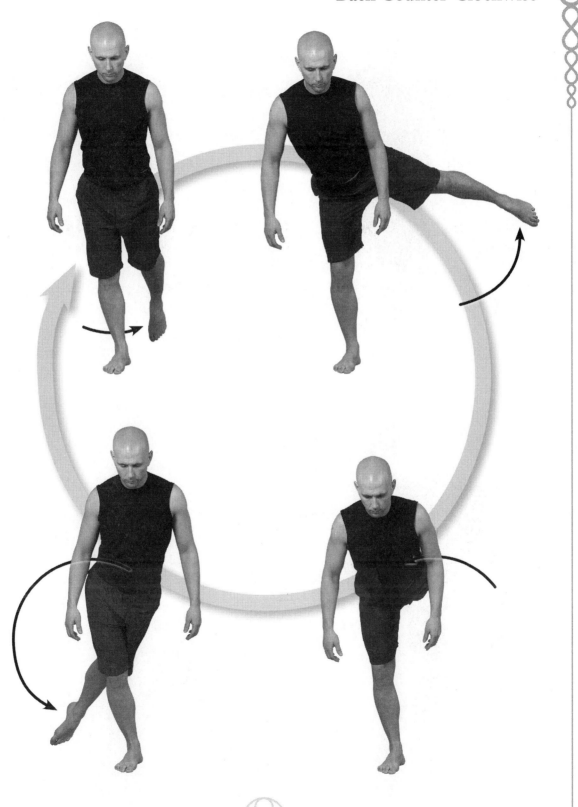

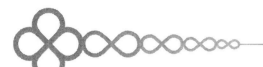

CIRCLES
Inside Clockwise

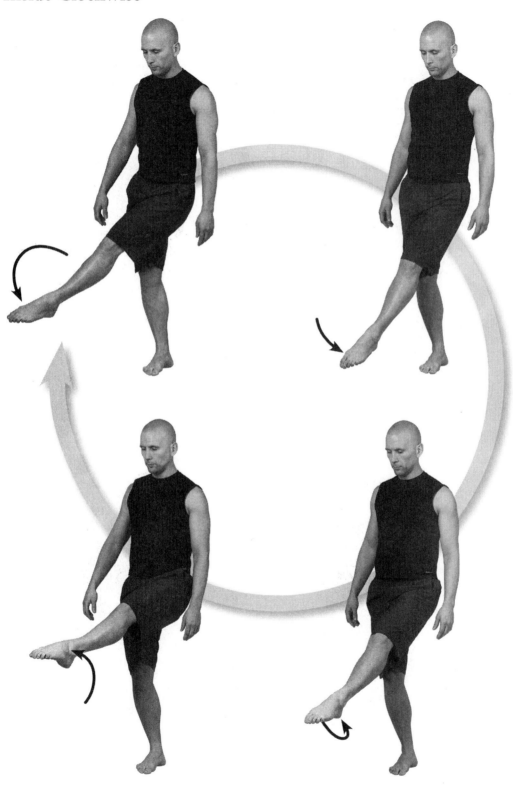

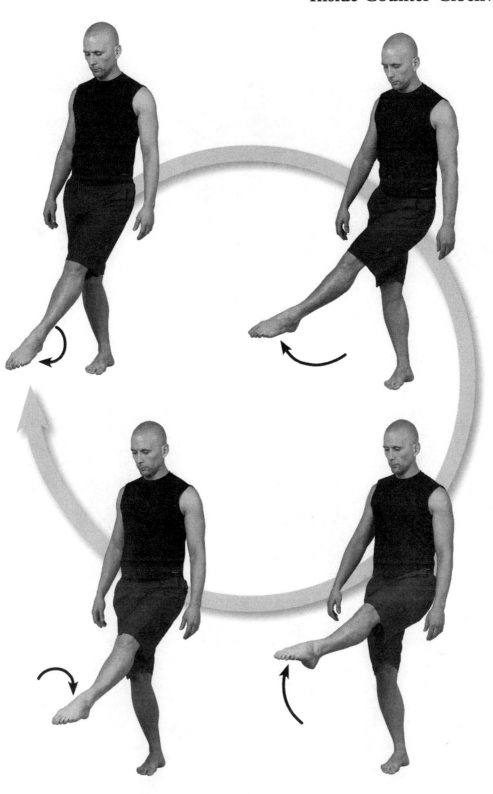

CIRCLES
Outside Clockwise

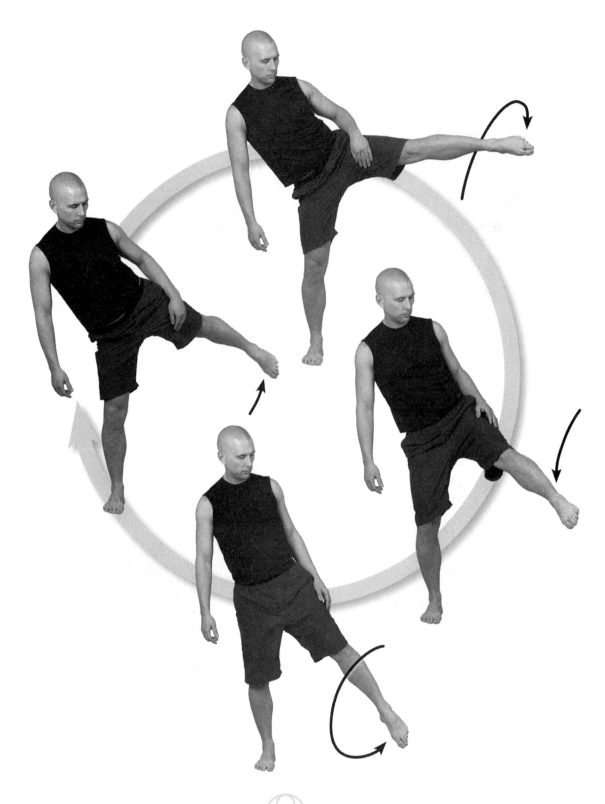

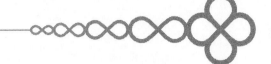

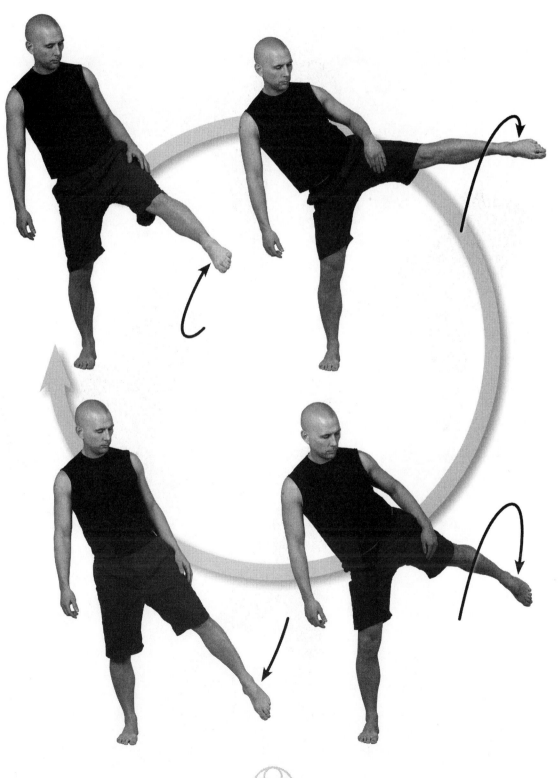

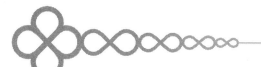

INFINITIES
Front – Back

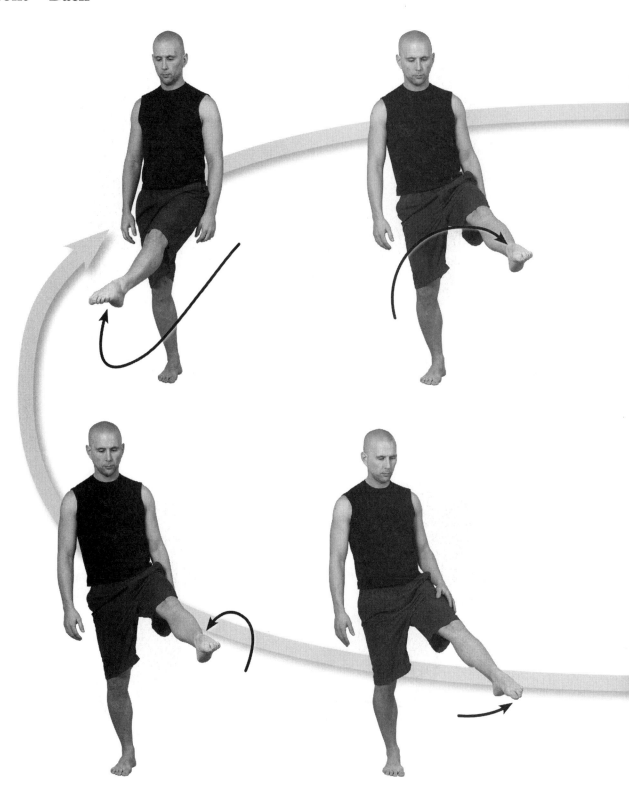

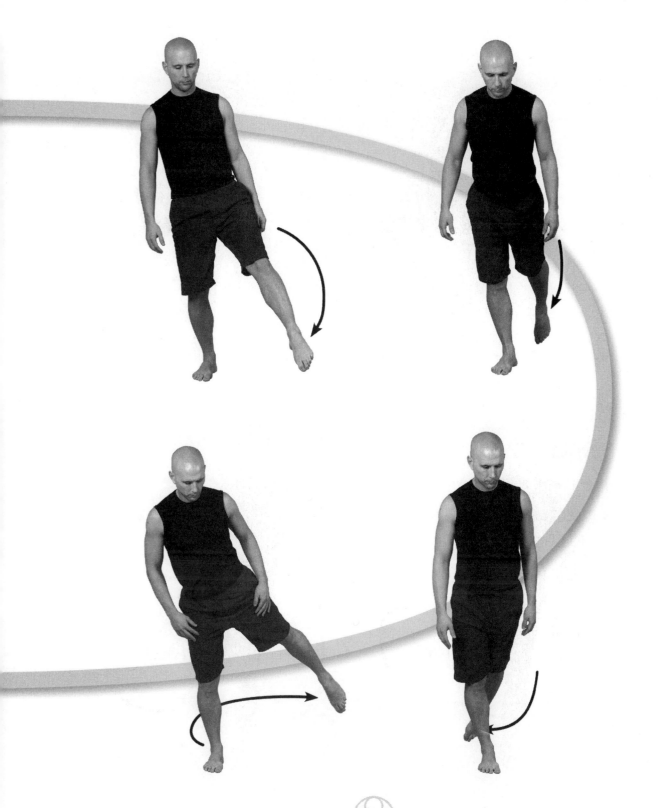

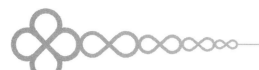

INFINITIES

Back – Front

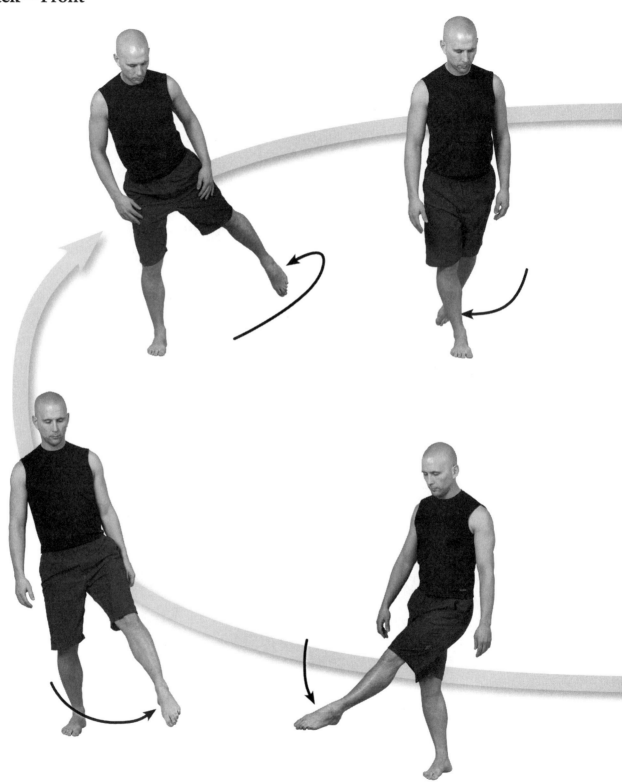

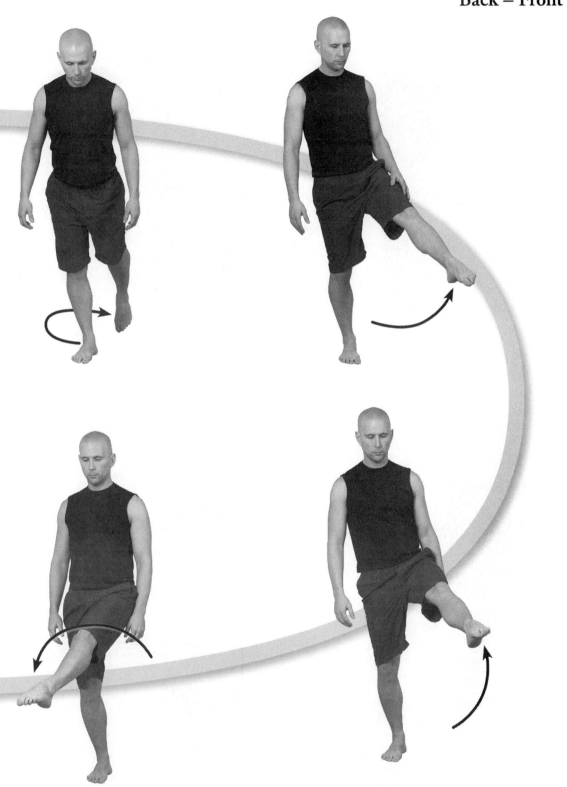

INFINITIES
Inside – Outside

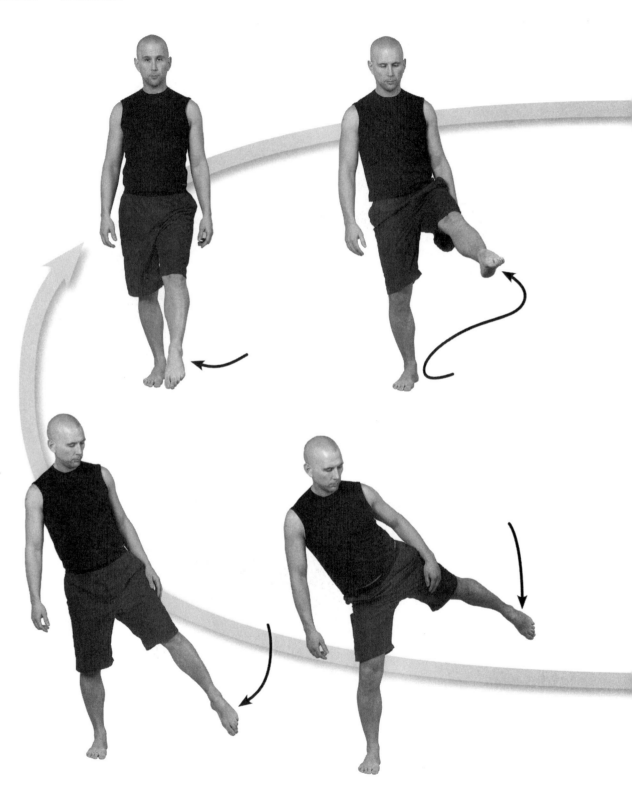

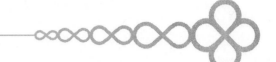

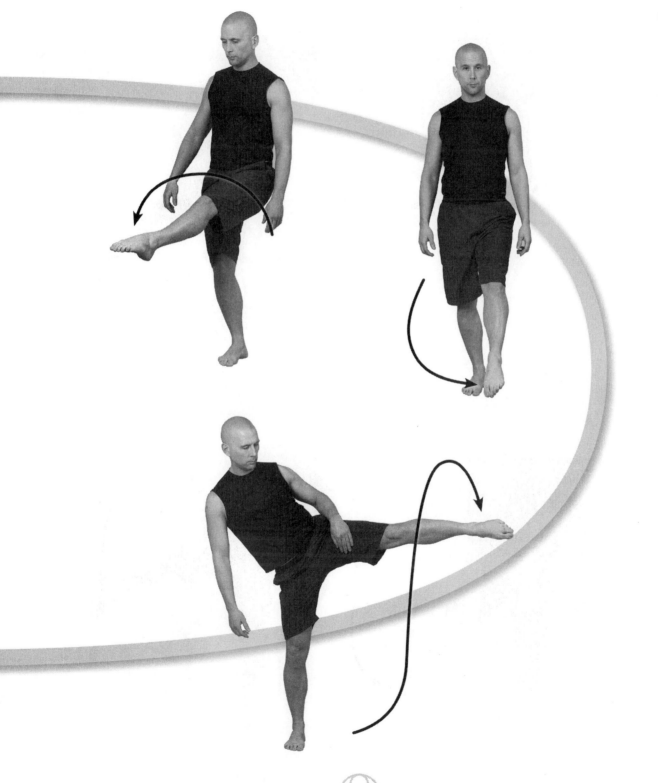

INFINITIES
Outside – Inside

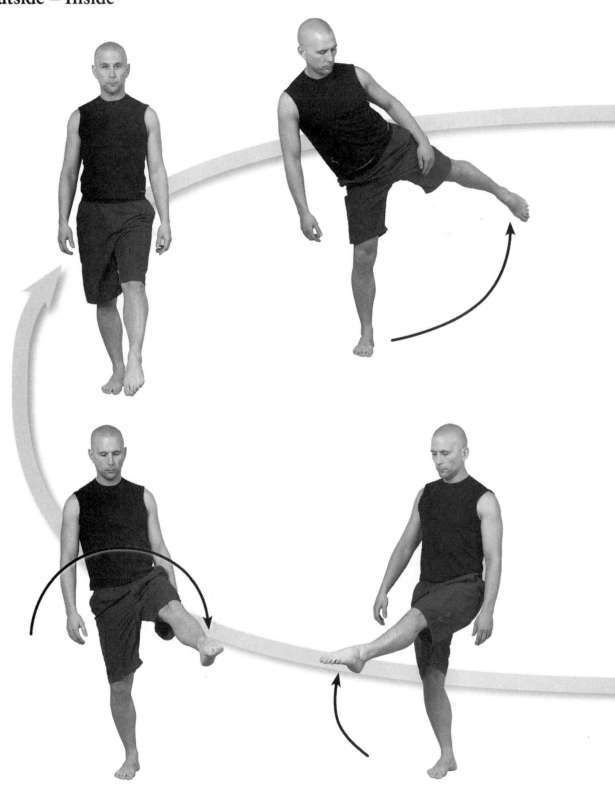

INFINITIES
Outside – Inside

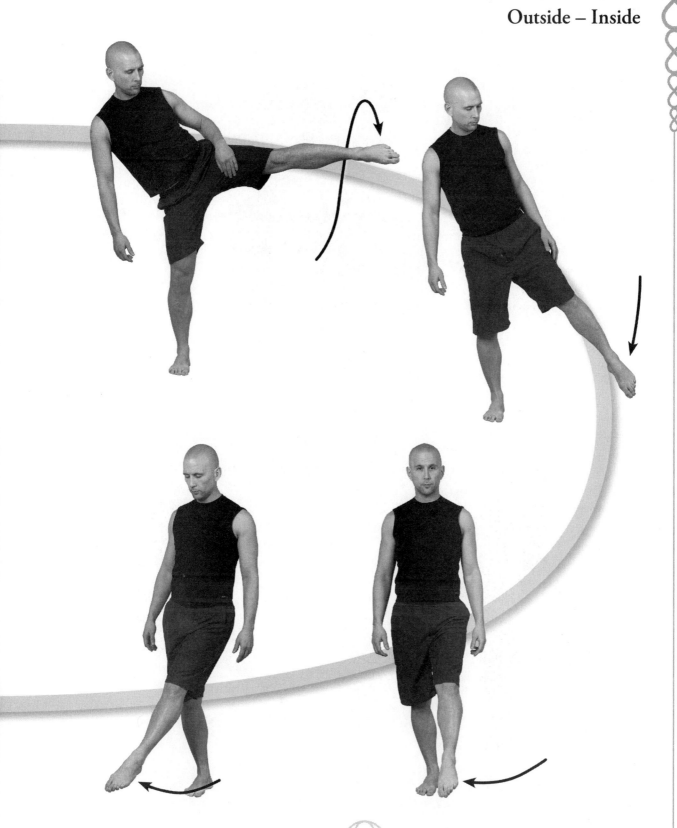

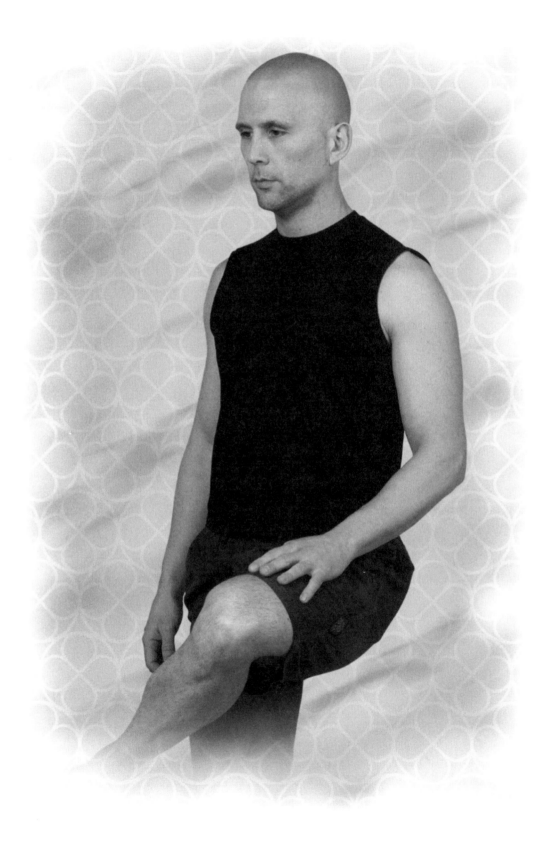

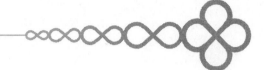

Knees & Legs

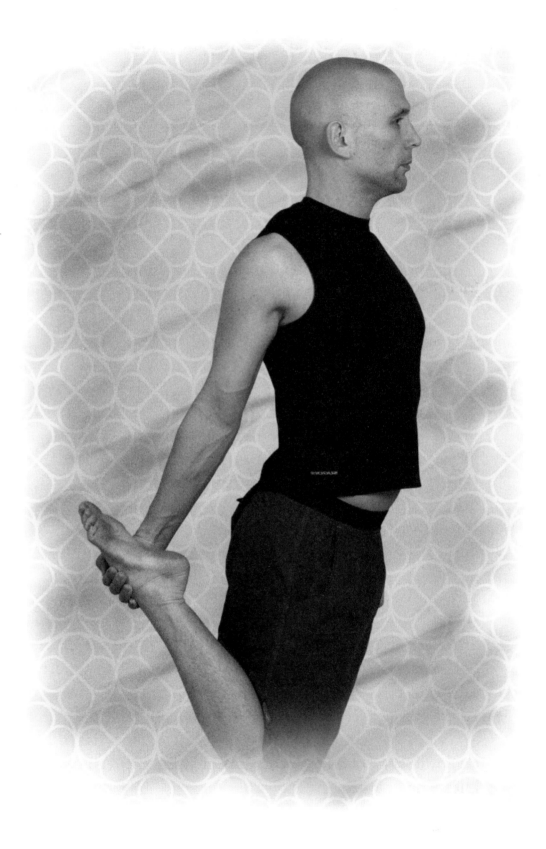

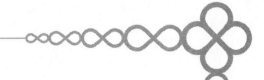

When not Free to Move from lack of prehabilitative movement due to stress, trauma, fear, overuse, underuse, or misuse, the following issues may result:

- Osteoarthritis
- Knee pain
- Iliotibial (IT) band friction syndrome
- Hamstring injuries
- Patellofemoral pain syndrome
- Plica syndrome
- Chondromalacia
- Meniscal injury
- Chronic compartment syndrome
- Shin splints

Common mental and emotional issues faced as a result of area not being Free to Move:

- Pride and ego can be too great
- Fear of failure over moving forward with life
- Feeling like you have to kneel down in subjugation
- Feeling a lack of foundation
- Feeling like your legs are giving out

Common organ referral affecting sensory-motor function of the area:

- There are no organs that refer pain directly to the knees; however, patients with kidney issues will sometimes report achy knees.
- While it is not technically organ referral, sometimes a lower back or pelvic problem (such as a herniated disc in the lower back or a nerve entrapment syndrome) can cause knee pain.

Knee/leg mobility that will help you become Free to Move again:

43. Ranges
   a. Forward Bend
   b. Standing King Dancer
   c. Shinbox
   d. Pigeon

44. Circles
   a. Front Clockwise and Counter-Clockwise
   b. Back Clockwise and Counter-Clockwise

45. Infinities
   a. Forward – Backward
   b. Backward – Forward
   c. Bottom – Top
   d. Top – Bottom
   e. Side Clockwise and Counter-Clockwise
   f. Rear Clockwise and Counter-Clockwise

46. Clovers
   a. Inside – outside – top – bottom – front – back

Forward Bend

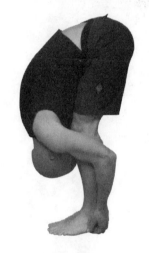

Standing King Dancer

Shinbox

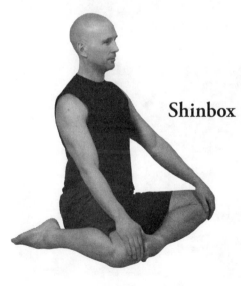

Pigeon

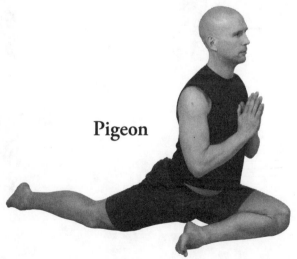

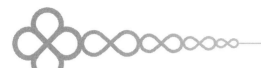

CIRCLES
Front Clockwise

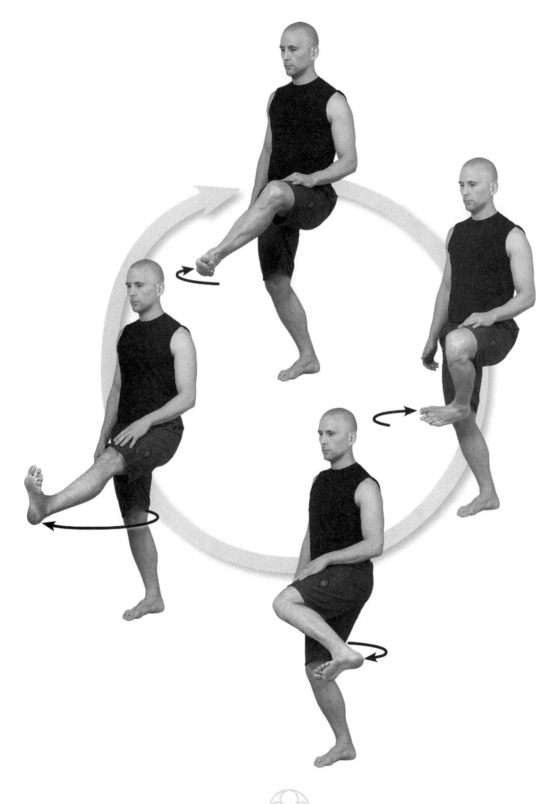

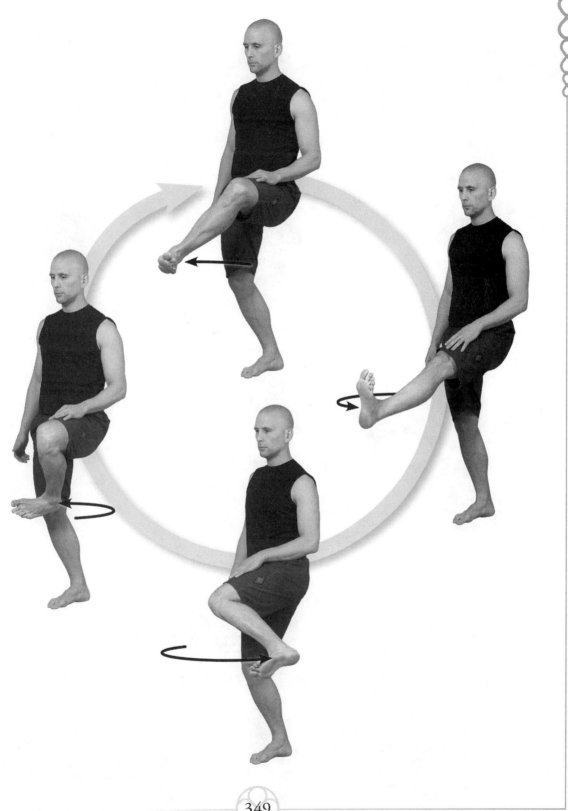

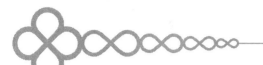

CIRCLES
Back Clockwise

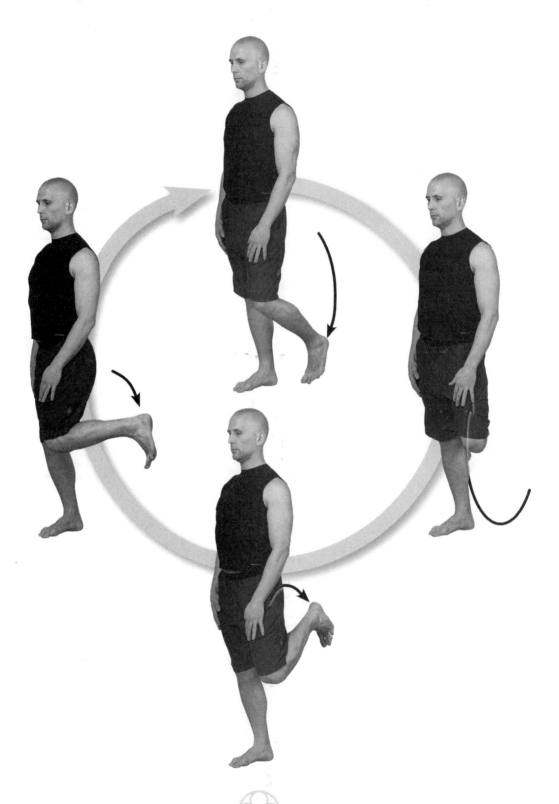

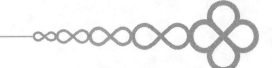

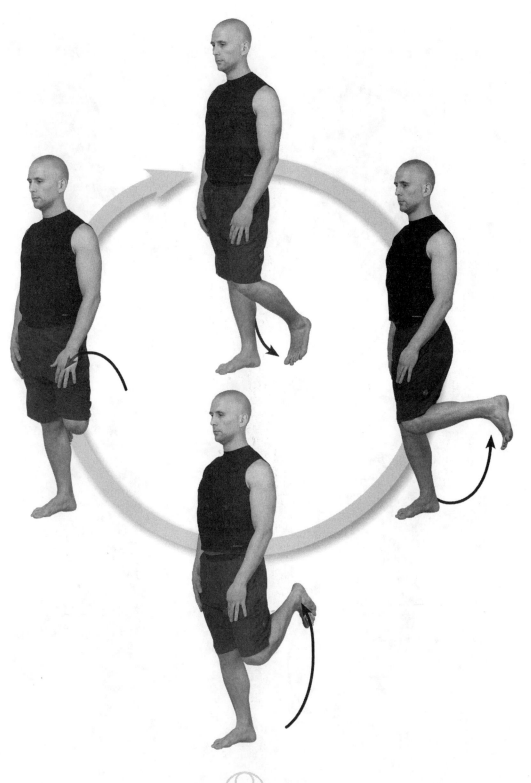

INFINITIES
Forward – Backward

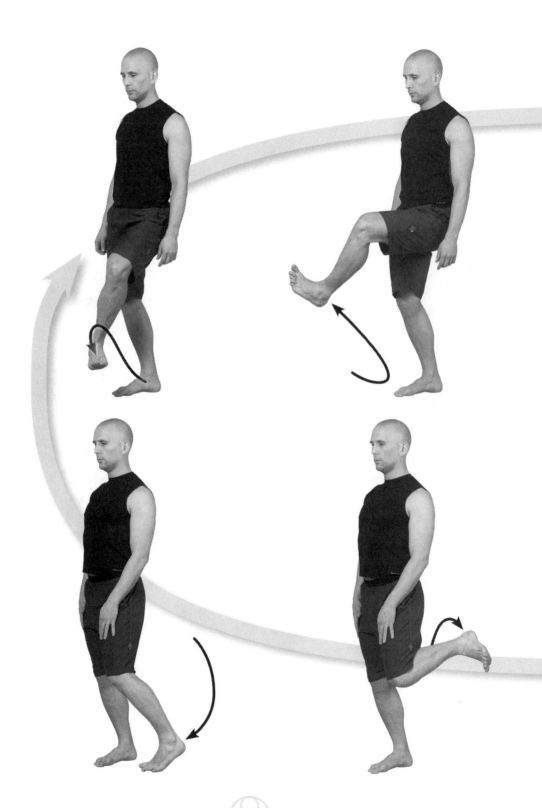

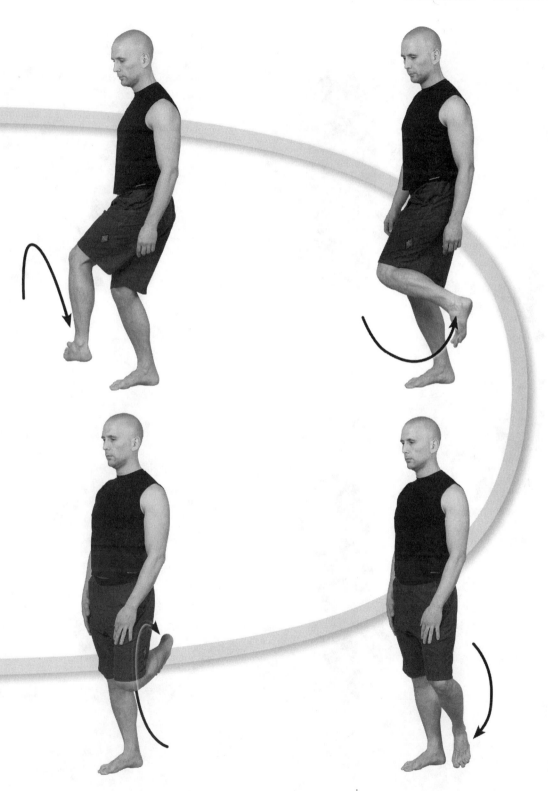

INFINITIES
Backward – Forward

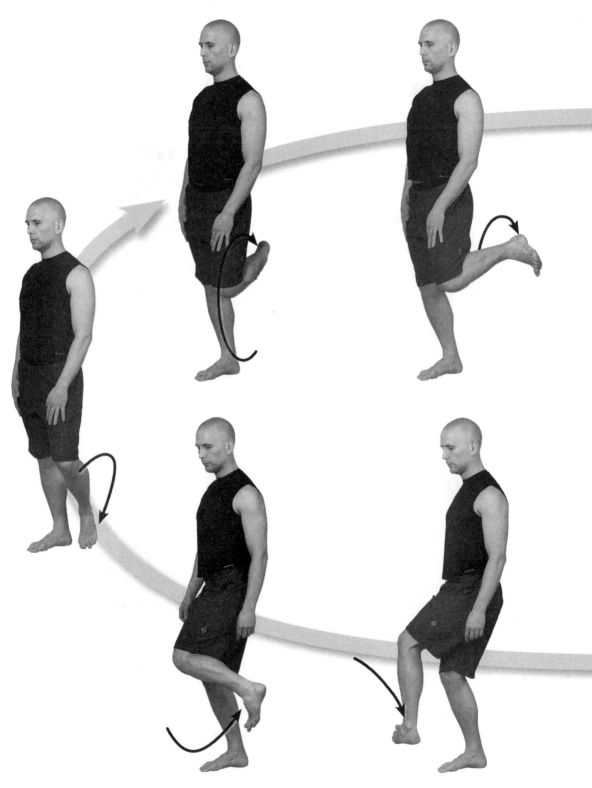

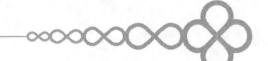

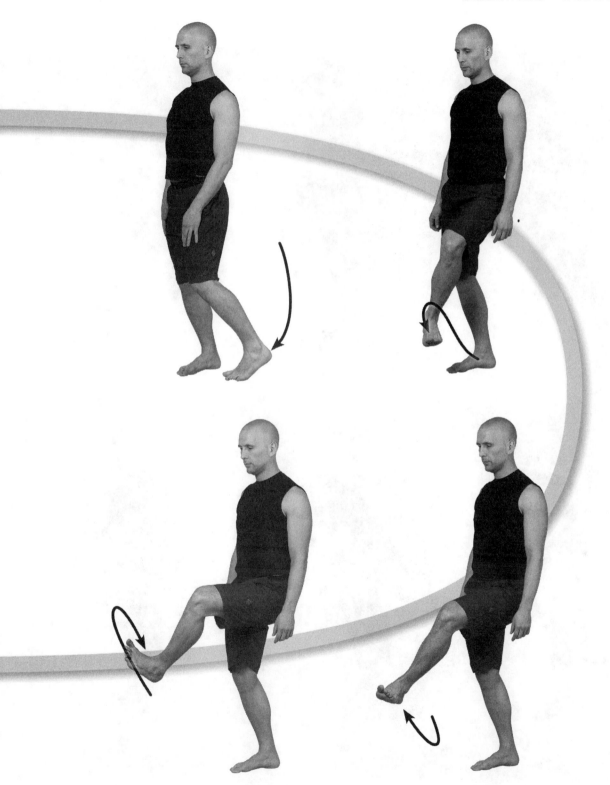

INFINITIES
Bottom – Top

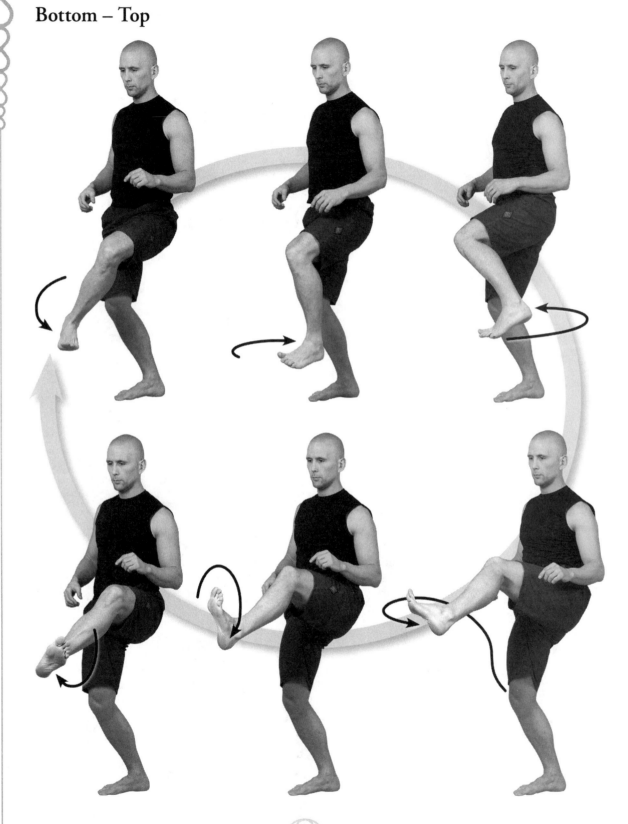

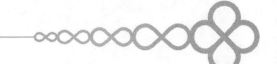

INFINITIES
Top – Bottom

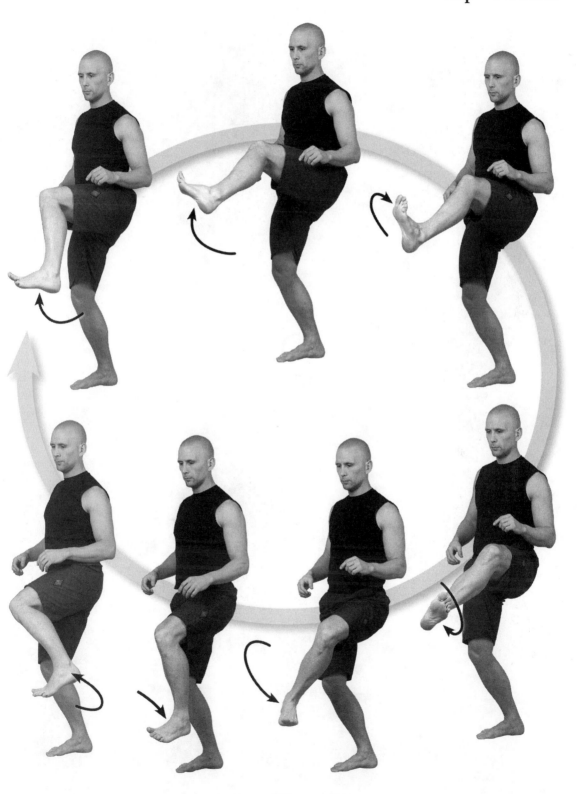

INFINITIES
Side Clockwise

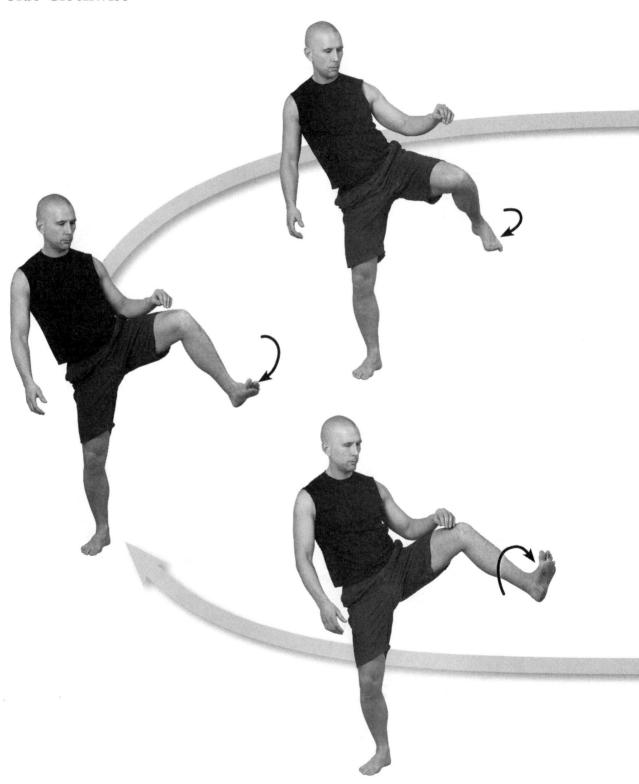

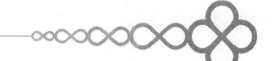

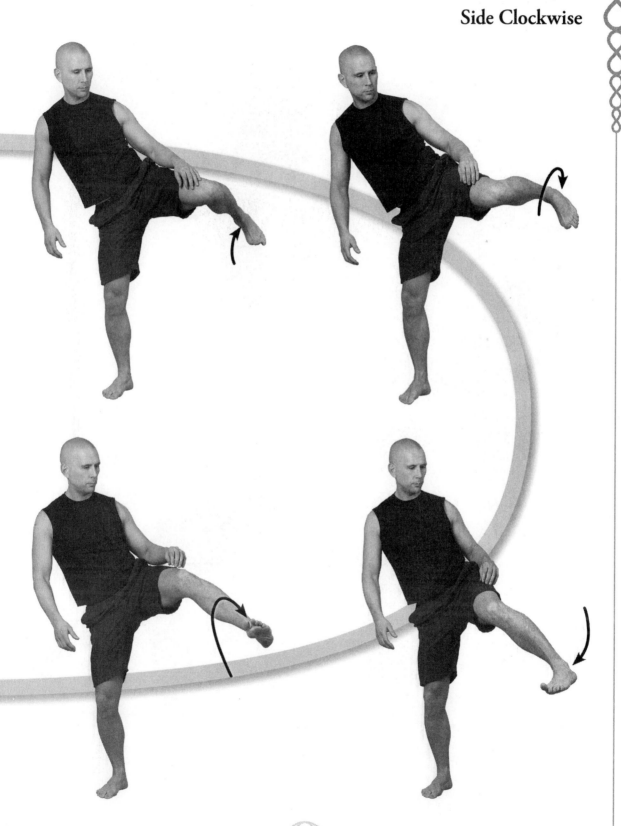

INFINITIES
Side Counter-Clockwise

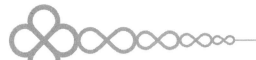
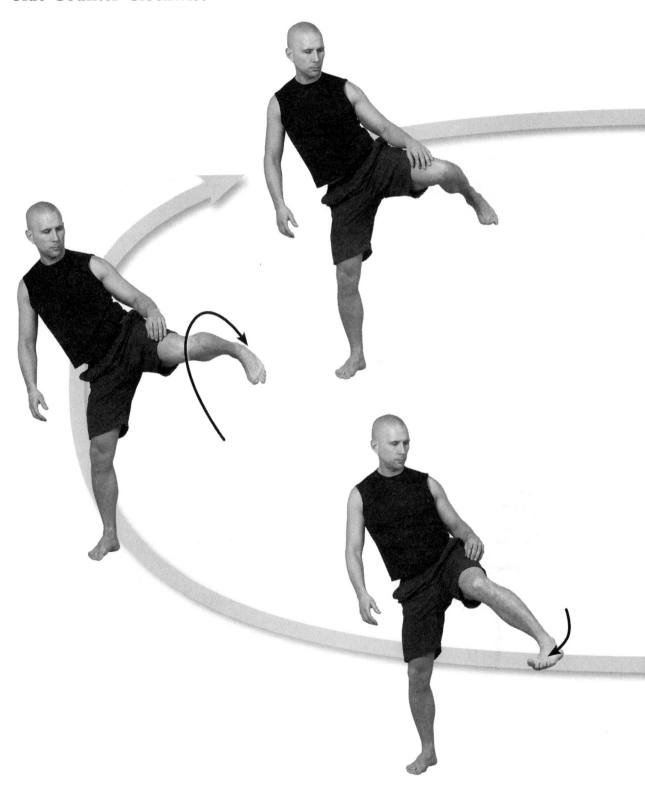

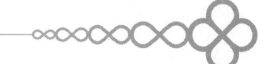

INFINITIES
Side Counter-Clockwise

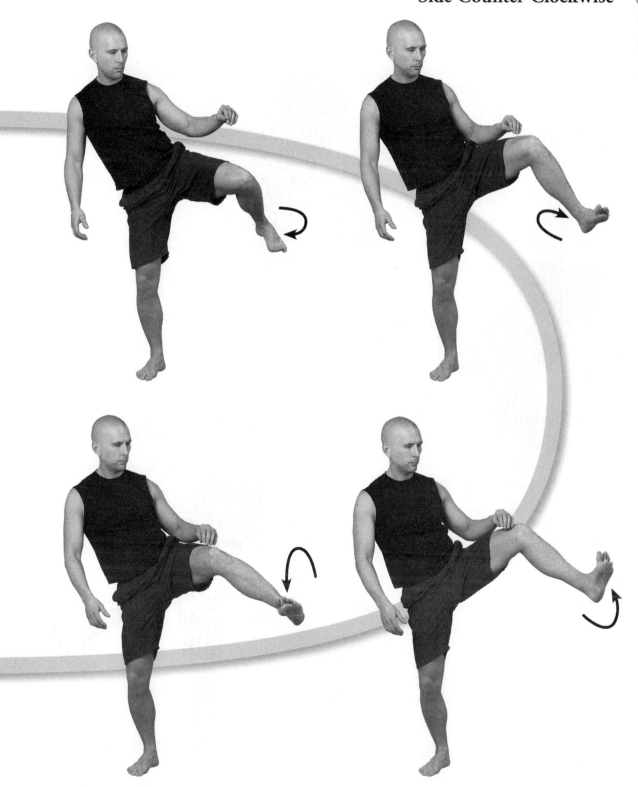

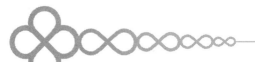

INFINITIES
Rear Clockwise

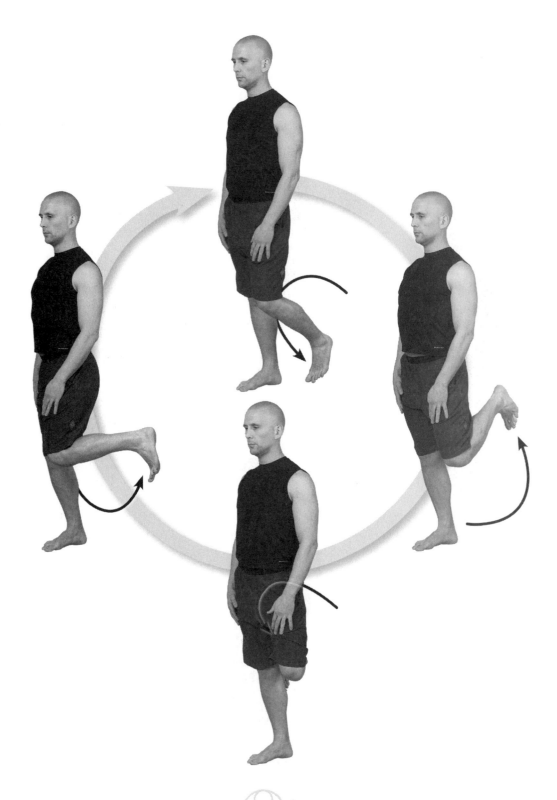

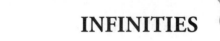

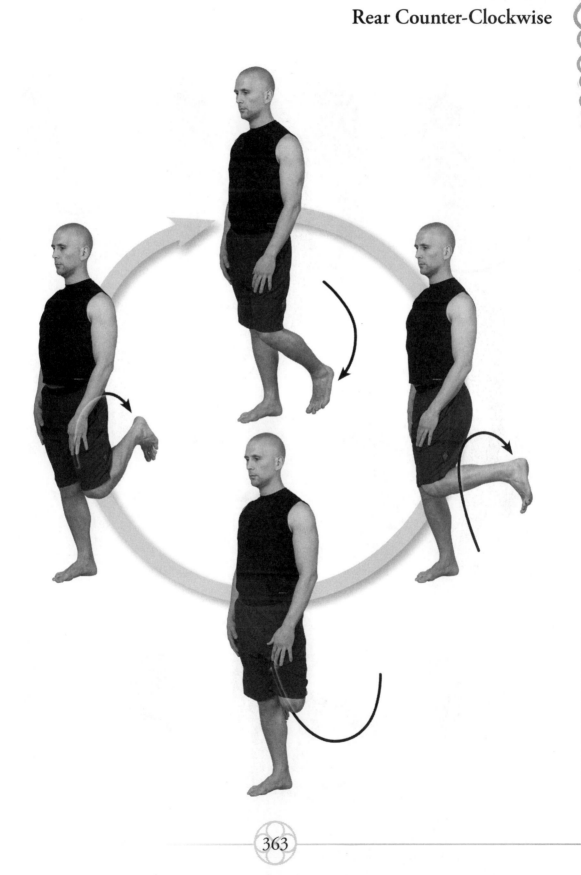

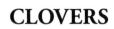

CLOVERS

Inside – outside – top – bottom – front – back

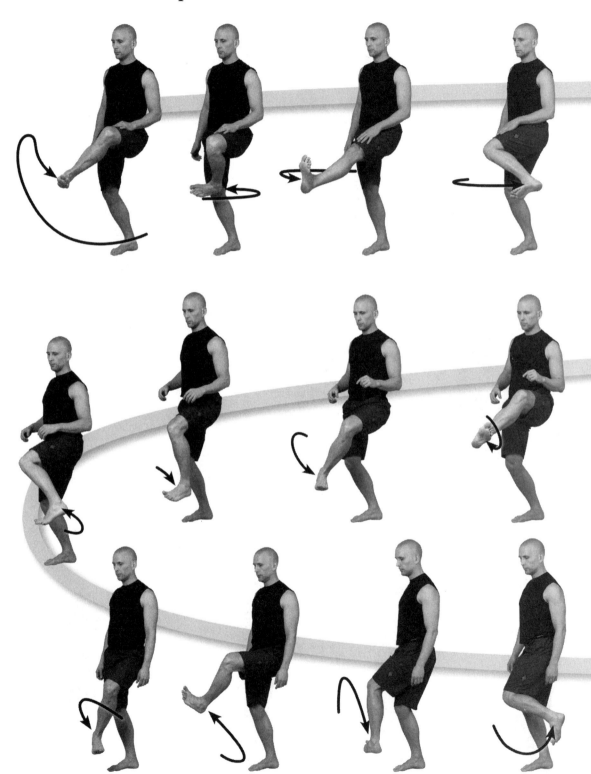

CLOVERS
Inside – outside – top – bottom – front – back

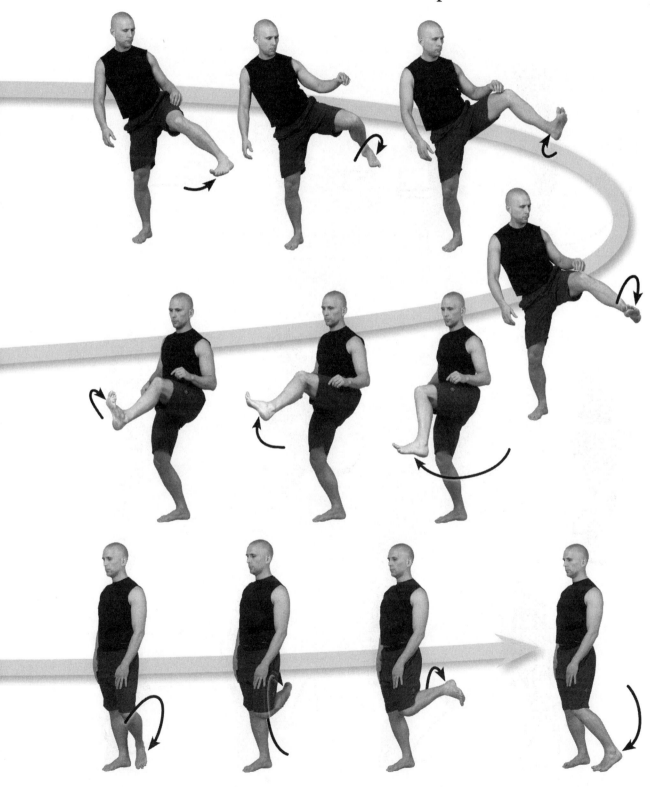

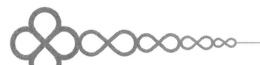

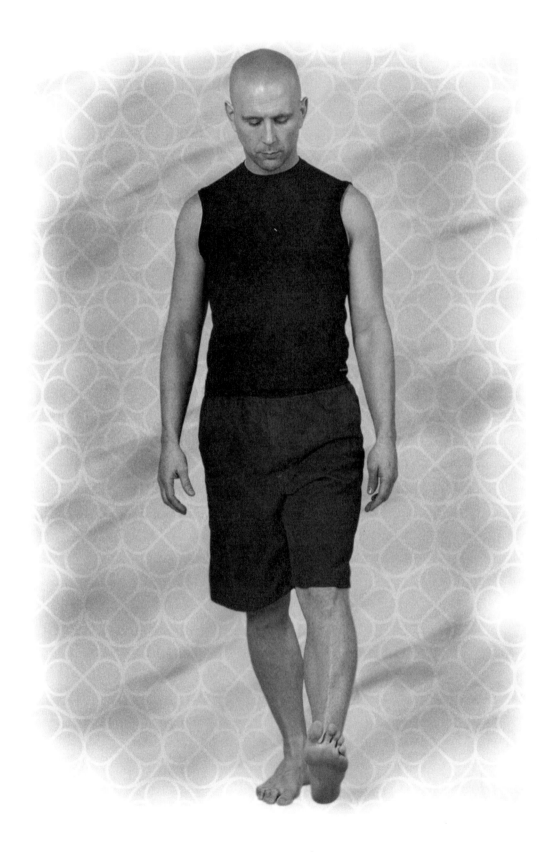

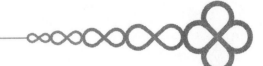

Ankles
Feet
Toes

When not Free to Move from lack of prehabilitative movement due to stress, trauma, fear, overuse, underuse, or misuse, the following issues may result:

- Osteoarthritis
- Achilles tendonitis
- Plantar fasciitis
- Heel spur
- Stress fracture
- Turf toe

Common mental and emotional issues faced as a result of area not being Free to Move:

- Guilt
- Fear of the future
- Not wanting to step forward in life
- Letting minor details prevent you from moving forward
- Feeling like you don't have the footing, a foot to stand on

Common organ referral affecting sensory-motor function of the area:

- There are no organs that refer pain directly to the ankles, feet, or toes.
- While it is not technically organ referral, sometimes a lower back or pelvic problem (such as a herniated disc in the lower back or nerve entrapment syndrome) can cause pain in the ankles, feet, and toes.

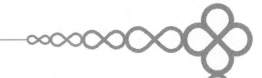

Mobility that will help you become Free to Move again:

47. **Ranges**
    a. Toe Point
    b. Pull Toes to Shin
    c. Tilt Inside
    d. Tilt Outside

48. **Circles**
    a. Point – inside – pull – outside
    b. Point – outside – pull – inside
    c. Foot Curl
    d. Foot Roll

49. **Infinities**
    a. Outside – point – inside – outside – pull – inside
    b. Inside – point – outside – inside – pull – outside
    c. Point – inside – pull – point – outside – pull
    d. Pull – inside – point – pull – outside – point

50. **Diagonal infinities**
    a. Point – inside – outside – pull – point
    b. Pull – outside – inside – point – pull
    c. Point – outside – inside – pull – point
    d. Pull – inside – outside – point – pull

51. **Clovers**
    a. Point – inside – outside – point – pull – outside
       – inside – pull
    b. Pull – inside – outside – pull – point – outside
       – inside – point

RANGES

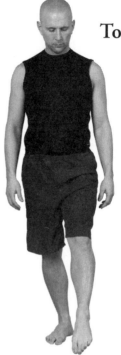

Toe Point

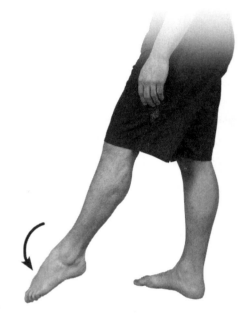

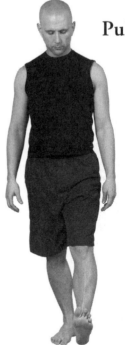

Pull Toes to Shin

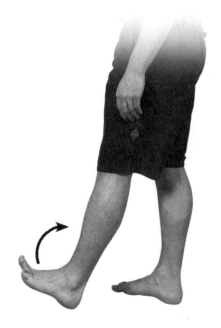

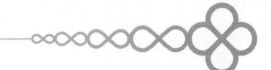

Tilt Inside

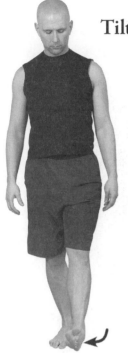

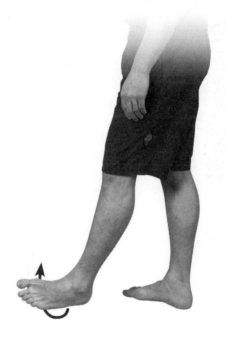

Tilt Outside

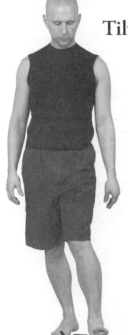

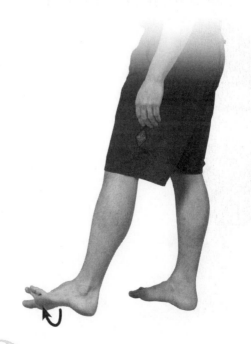

CIRCLES

Point – inside – pull – outside

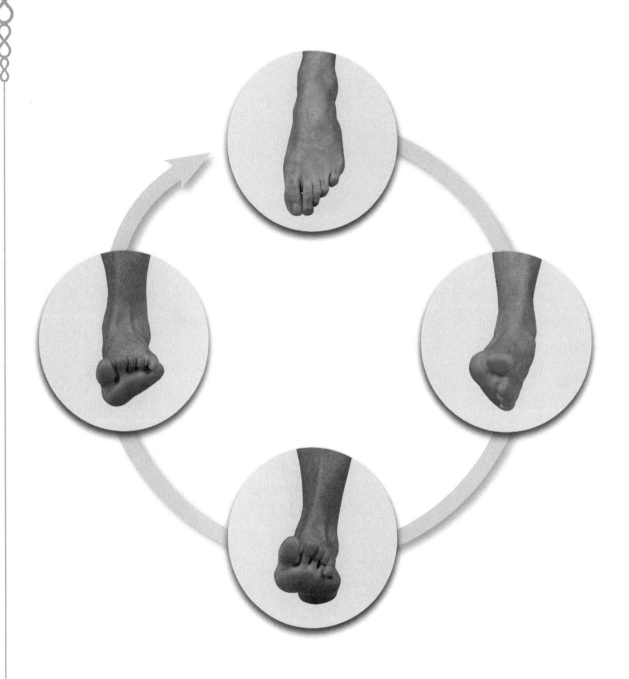

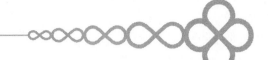

CIRCLES
Point – outside – pull – inside

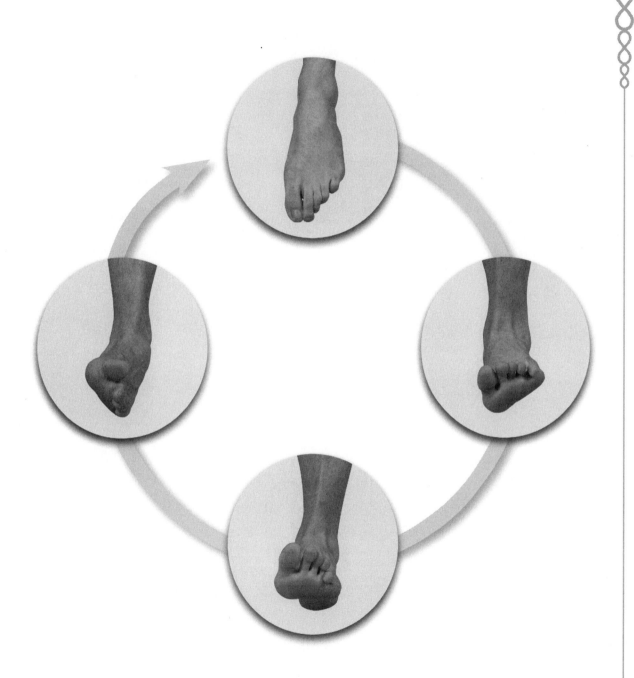

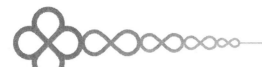

CIRCLES
Foot Curl

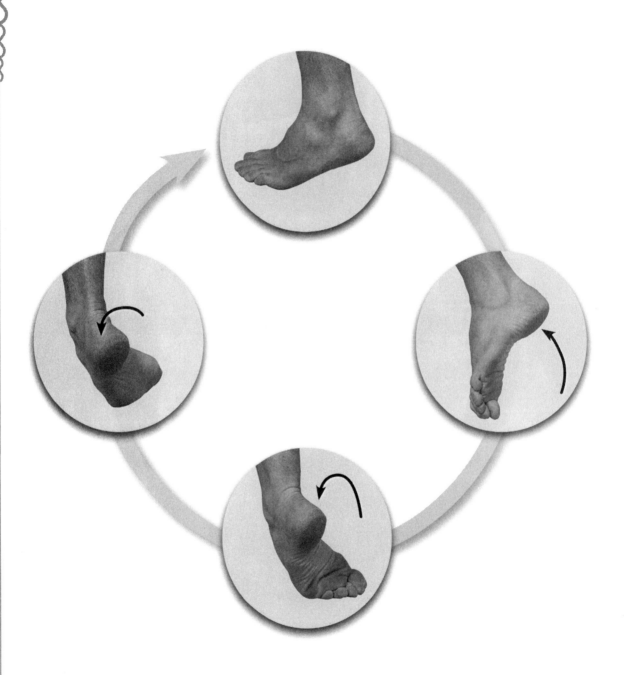

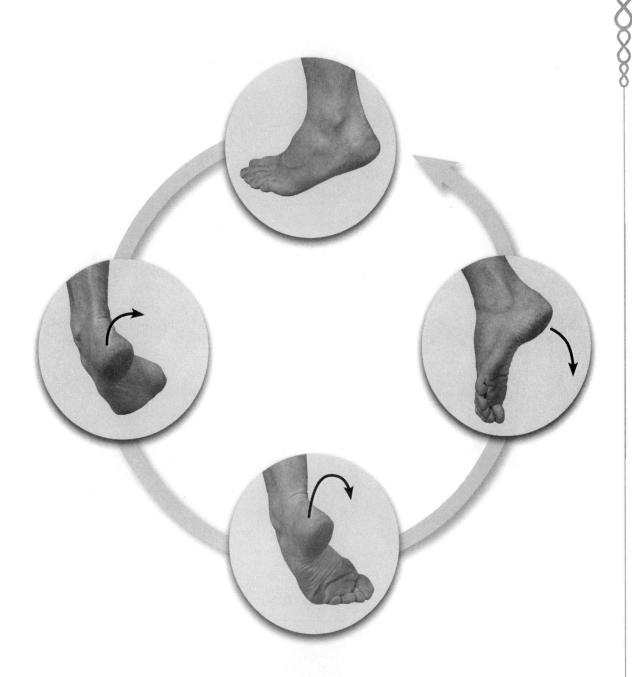

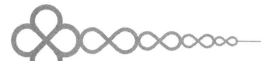

INFINITIES

Outside – point – inside – outside – pull – inside

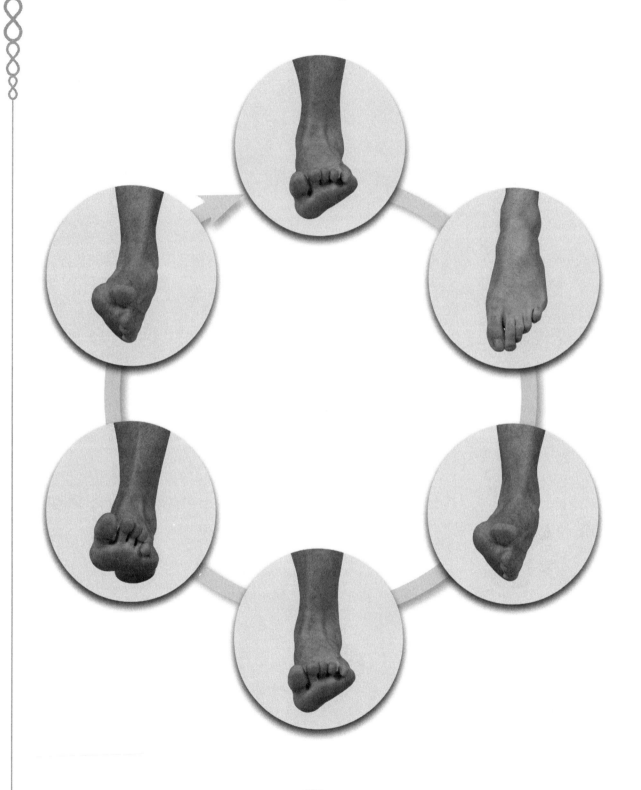

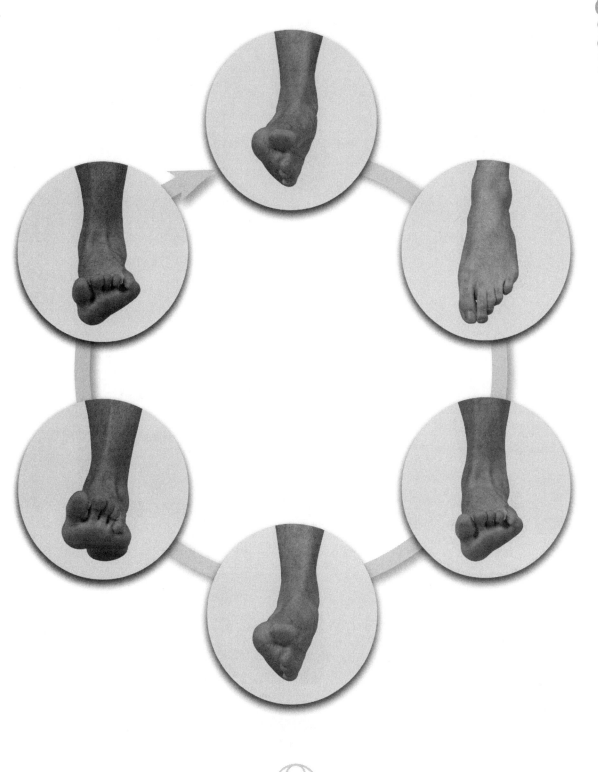

INFINITIES

Point – inside – pull – point – outside – pull

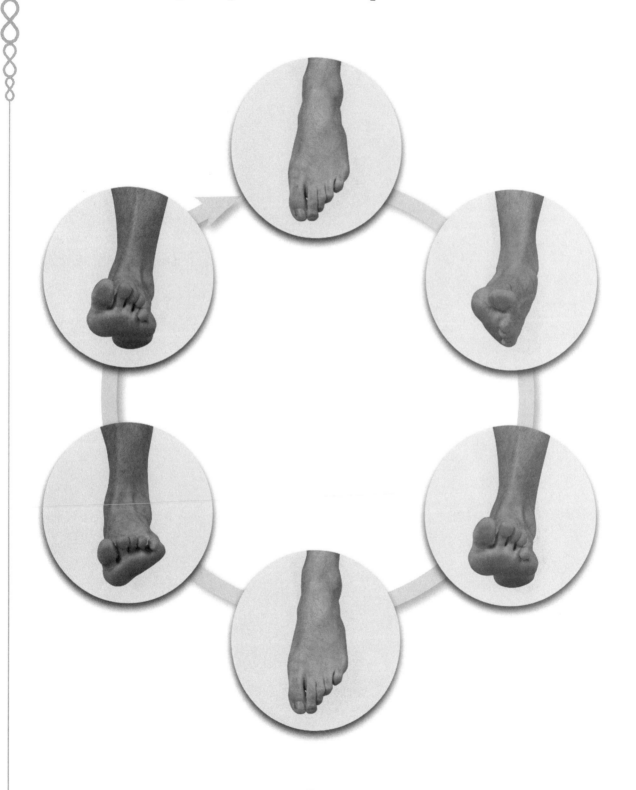

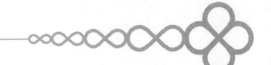

INFINITIES
Pull – inside – point – pull – outside – point

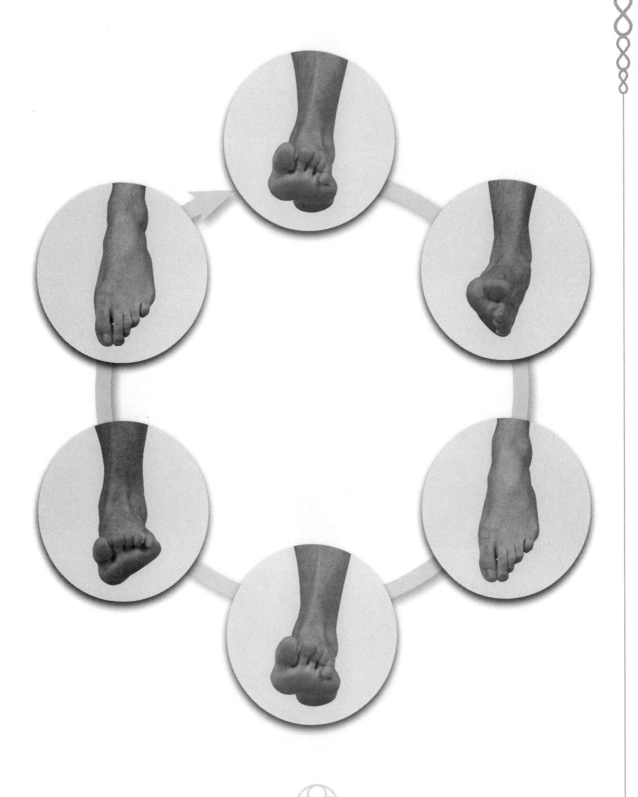

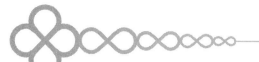

DIAGONAL INFINITIES

Point – inside – outside – pull – point

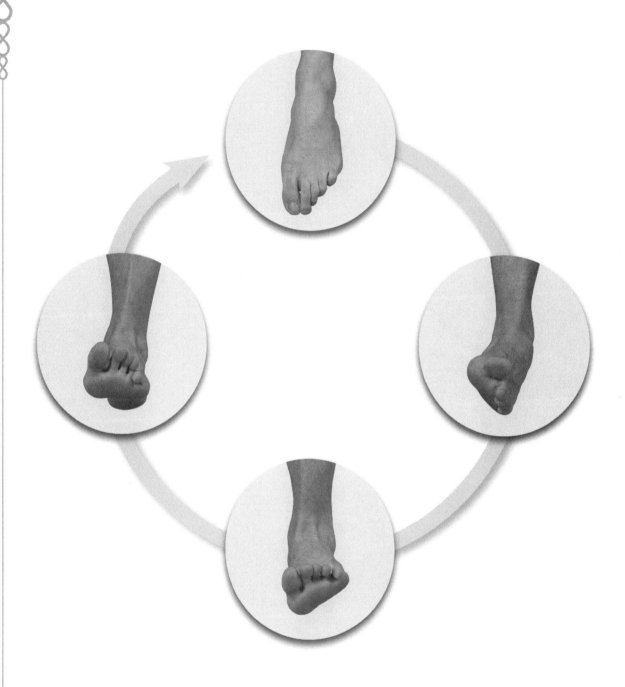

DIAGONAL INFINITIES
Pull – outside – inside – point – pull

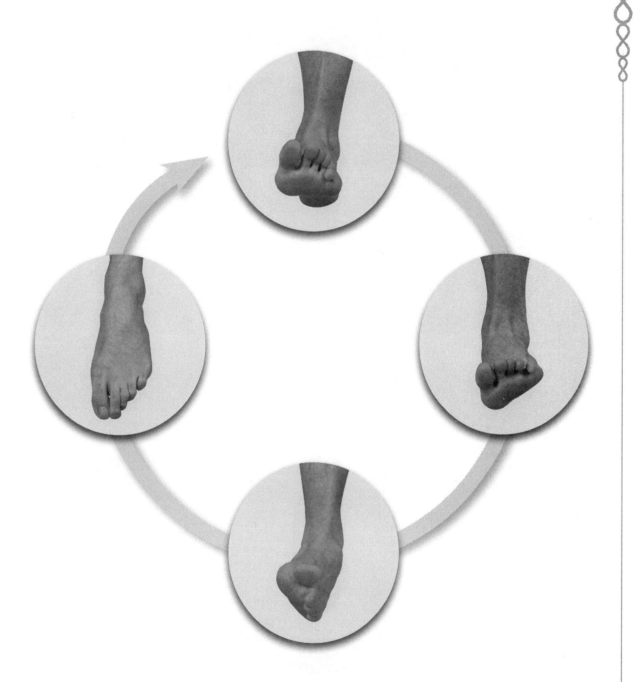

DIAGONAL INFINITIES

Point – outside – inside – pull – point

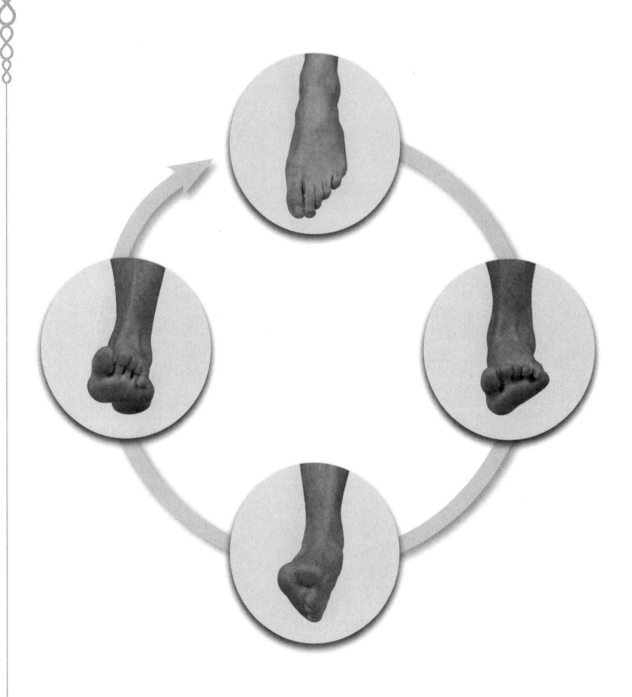

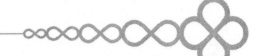

DIAGONAL INFINITIES
Pull – inside – outside – point – pull

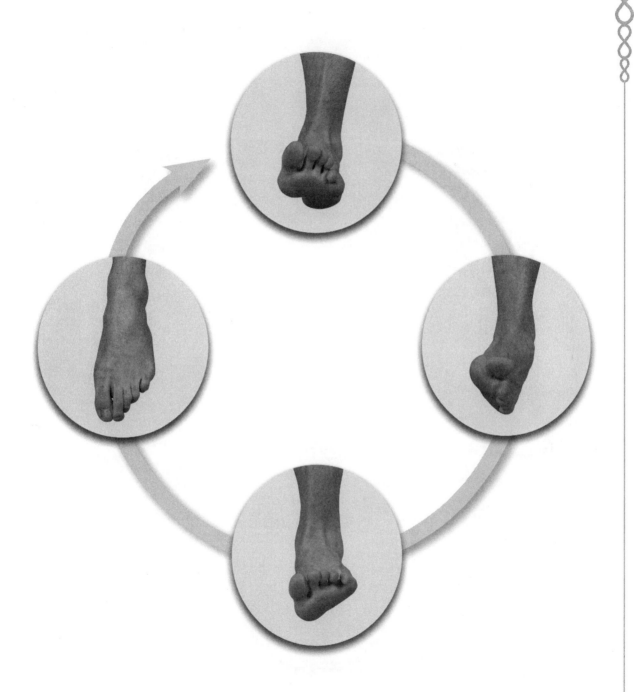

CLOVERS

Point – inside – outside – point – pull – outside – inside – pull

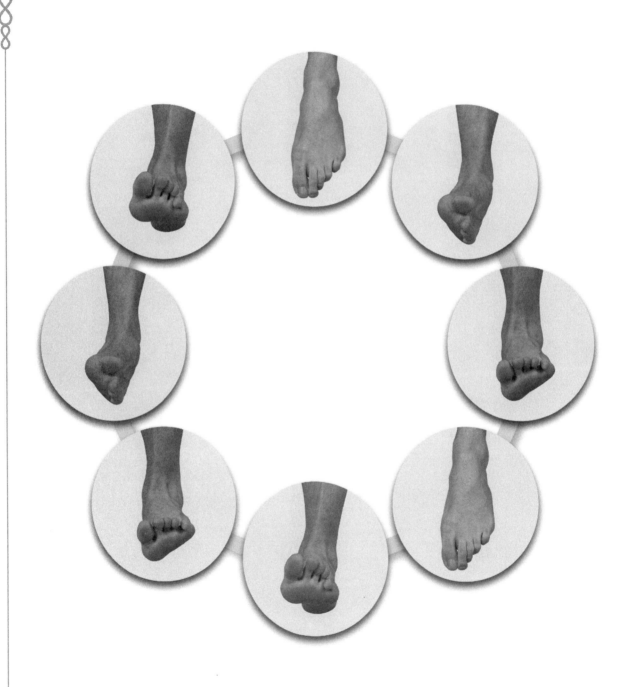

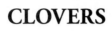

CLOVERS

Pull – inside – outside – pull – point – outside – inside – point

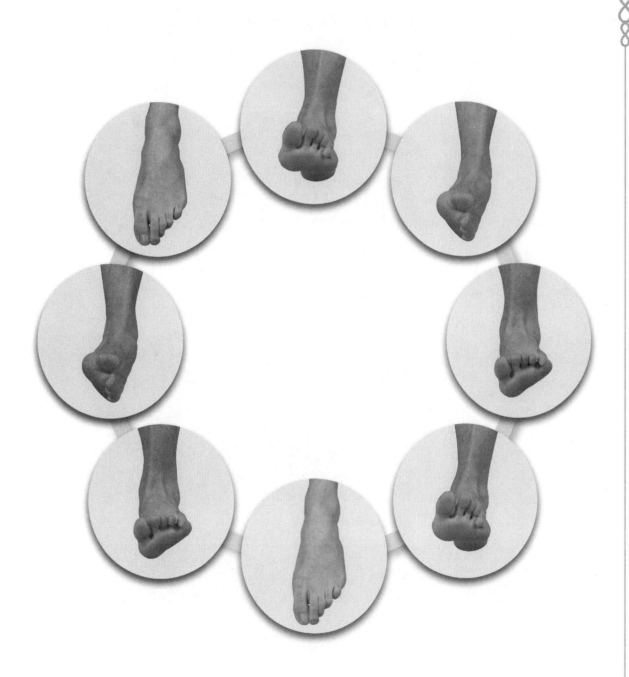

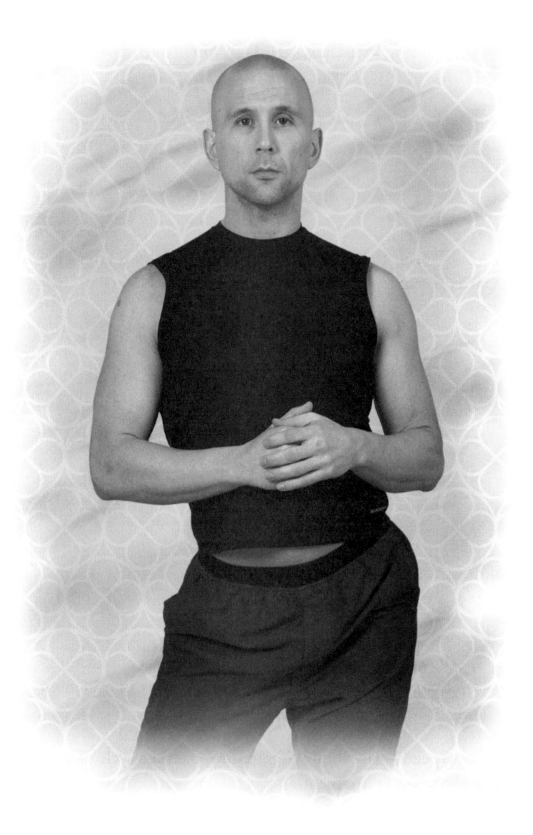

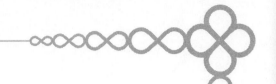

Final Word

WHAT IS YOUR PRIMARY FITNESS ATTRIBUTE?

The conventional strength and conditioning community defines the array of foundational fitness attributes as follows:

1. **Cardiovascular/Respiratory Endurance** – The ability of the body's systems to gather process and deliver oxygen.

2. **Stamina** – The ability of the body's systems to process, deliver, store and use energy.

3. **Strength** – The ability of a muscular unit or combination of muscular units to apply force.

4. **Flexibility** – The ability to maximize the range of motion at a given joint.

5. **Power** – The ability of a muscular unit or combination of muscular units to apply maximum force in minimum time.

6. **Speed** – The ability to minimize the time cycle of a repeated movement.

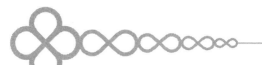
7. **Coordination** – The ability to combine several distinct movement patterns into a singular distinct movement.

8. **Agility** – The ability to minimize transition time from one movement pattern to another.

9. **Balance** – The ability to control the placement of the body's center of gravity in relation to its support base.

10. **Accuracy** – The ability to control movement in a given direction or at a given intensity

Each of these 10 attributes requires one essential characteristic in order to function. None of these attributes mean anything without this most a priori virtue of fitness: **mobility.**

MOBILITY IS YOUR VERY EXISTENCE

- Mobility is the prime requisite of strength and power. Without mobility, the muscle cannot maximally contract. (Even "isometric" strength training is internal movement against an immovable external resistance.)

- Mobility is the foundation of sports and athletic performance. It enables speed, agility, coordination and accuracy. The less mobile you are, the slower, less agile, less coordinated, and less accurate you will be.

- Mobility defines range of motion and flexibility. You cannot have range or flexibility without it.

- Without Mobility you cannot acquire or refine new skills.

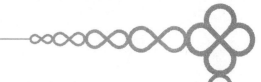

- Diminish mobility and you increase pain! The body despises immobility, and it sends you persistent messages in the form of discomfort or pain when you refuse to move.

- Without mobility, your lungs cannot breathe, your heart cannot pump, and your blood cannot circulate effectively. Without mobility you cannot lubricate nor deliver nutrition to your connective tissue. You are literally committing daily suicide without mobility!

- Decrease your mobility and you accelerate the aging process. Remember, we are as young as our mobility!

Twelve years ago I coined the terms "joint mobility" and "circular strength" to refer to this most critical attribute of fitness upon which all others are built. Over the course of those twelve years, while I've been traveling the world speaking to strength and conditioning, fitness, yoga, wellness, academic and clinical organizations, I've finally seen Mobility elevated to its rightful place in the hierarchy of fundamental fitness attributes.

To regain and refine your mobility, to become "Free to Move," start practicing the exercises within these pages. If you need a three-dimensional visualization of the movements, go to www.Intu-Flow.com and get the Intu-Flow Longevity System DVDs — the original, most comprehensive and most effective joint mobility program ever created.

The benefits are astronomical! Mobility is life!

MOVE IT OR LOSE IT!

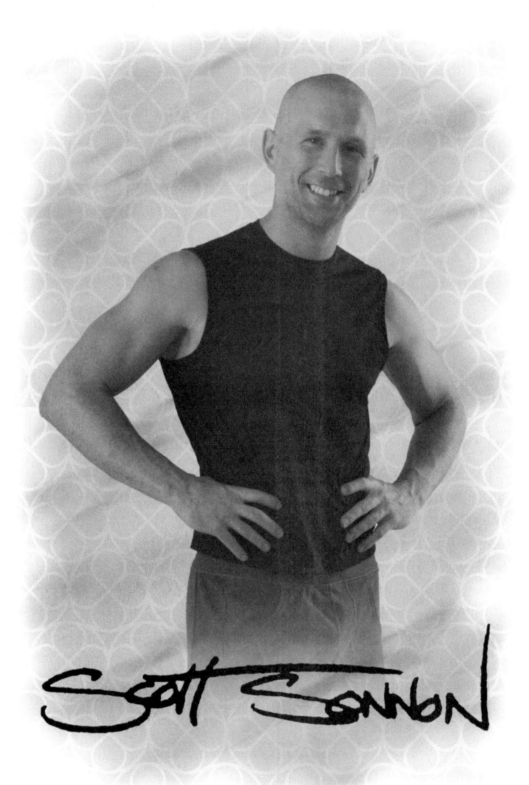